T0321155

Clinics in Developmental Medicine

THE EPILEPSY-APHASIA SPECTRUM
FROM LANDAU-KLEFFNER SYNDROME TO
ROLANDIC EPILEPSY

The Epilepsy-Aphasia Spectrum From Landau-Kleffner Syndrome to Rolandic Epilepsy

by

THIERRY DEONNA
Pediatric Neurology and Neurorehabilitation Unit, Department of
Pediatric Medicine and Surgery, Lausanne University Hospital,
(Centre Hospitalier Universitaire Vaudois), Switzerland

and

ELIANE ROULET-PEREZ
Pediatric Neurology and Neurorehabilitation Unit, Lausanne
University Hospital (Centre Hospitalier Universitaire Vaudois); Faculty
of Biology and Medicine, University of Lausanne, Switzerland

with contributions from

XAVIER DE TIÈGE, SERGE GOLDMAN and PATRICK VAN BOGAERT,
Laboratoire de Cartographie fonctionnelle du Cerveau, The ULB
Neuroscience Institute, Université libre de Bruxelles, Belgium

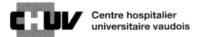
Centre hospitalier
universitaire vaudois

2016
Mac Keith Press

© 2016 Mac Keith Press
6 Market Road, London, N7 9PW

Managing Director: Ann-Marie Halligan
Production Manager and Commissioning Editor: Udoka Ohuonu
Project Management: Lumina Datamatics

The views and opinions expressed herein are those of the authors and do not necessarily represent those of the publisher.

First published in this edition in 2016

British Library Cataloguing-in-Publication data
A catalogue record for this book is available from the British Library

Cover design: Hannah Rogers

ISBN: 978-1-909962-76-7

Typeset by Lumina Datamatics, Chennai, India

Printing managed by Jellyfish Solutions Ltd, UK

Mac Keith Press is supported by Scope

CONTENTS

AUTHORS' APPOINTMENTS

Xavier De Tiège   Associate Professor, Laboratoire de Cartographie fonctionnelle du Cerveau, The ULB Neuroscience Institute, Université libre de Bruxelles, Belgium

Thierry Deonna   Professor Emeritus of Child Neurology, Pediatric Neurology and Neurorehabilitation Unit, Department of Pediatric Medicine and Surgery, Lausanne University Hospital (Centre Hospitalier Universitaire Vaudois), Lausanne, Switzerland

Serge Goldman   Director, Laboratoire de Cartographie fonctionnelle du Cerveau, ULB Neuroscience Institute, Université libre de Bruxelles, Belgium

Eliane Roulet-Perez Head of the Pediatric Neurology and Neurorehabilitation Unit, Lausanne University Hospital (Centre Hospitalier Universitaire Vaudois); Professor of Paediatric Neurology, Faculty of Biology and Medicine, University of Lausanne, Lausanne, Switzerland

Patrick Van Bogaert Co-director, Laboratoire de Cartographie fonctionnelle du Cerveau, The ULB Neuroscience Institute, Université libre de Bruxelles, Belgium

FOREWORD

It is rare to find a book that one can recommend with equal enthusiasm to clinicians and researchers, but *The Epilepsy-Aphasia Spectrum; From Landau-kleffner syndrome to Rolandic Epilepsy* is just such a volume. The overarching topic–the relationship between childhood epilepsy and cognition, especially language–is a fascinating one that holds many intellectual puzzles. Why do some children deteriorate after a period of normal development, losing skills they once had? What is the relationship between the aphasia and the epilepsy—does one cause the other, or are they separate consequences of a common underlying cause? Can we predict which children will regain their lost skills?

There are several features of acquired epileptic aphasia that make these questions particularly difficult. Heterogeneity at both clinical and aetiological levels is a major challenge, especially given the rarity of these disorders, which can make it difficult to draw generalisations from a group of cases. Deonna and Roulet-Perez point out how an over-narrow conceptualisation of Landau–Kleffner syndrome (for which, I discovered, I was in part, unwittingly, responsible!) led to the neglect of research on children whose speech and language problems went beyond the classic picture of verbal auditory agnosia. They present a wealth of clinical case histories that show just how variable the presentation can be. Variability characterises not just the initial presentation but also the course of the disorder. Children can recover after a substantial regression only to regress again months or years later. Careful longitudinal studies can be helpful in studying the vexed question of the causal relationship between epilepsy and cognition, but it is clear that there can be a far more neurophysiological abnormality than may be evident from a simple observation of seizures. Drugs that control the seizures may leave language deficits untouched, and indeed may even make the condition worse.

This book notes the fluid boundaries between classic 'Landau–Kleffner syndrome' and other childhood epilepsies. It is noted that rolandic epilepsy has many features in common with Landau–Kleffner syndrome, but with a focus on the centro-temporal rather than posterior-temporal cortex.

In the midst of this scholarly account of the nature and manifestations of these epileptic syndromes, we never lose sight of the family and child whose lives can be turned upside down by a sudden change in cognition and behaviour. As Deonna and Roulet-Perez put it: 'How can a young human being cope with a prolonged loss of language while keeping otherwise preserved intellectual and emotional abilities and adapt without losing his essential self?' Chapters on drug treatment, surgery, and educational approaches are illustrated with carefully documented case histories, and there is a particularly thoughtful account of the benefits of sign language for many children with a verbal auditory agnosia. This book ends with some vivid first-hand accounts of the impact of language loss by adults who have grown up with Landau–Kleffner syndrome.

Dorothy Bishop
Professor, Department of Developmental Neuropsychology,
University of Oxford, UK

FOREWORD

The Landau–Kleffner syndrome (LKS) is not a common condition. There are, however, many reasons why a book should be devoted to it.

The diagnosis should come to mind when confronted by a child with comparatively mild epilepsy who has difficulty in understanding verbal requests to carry out non-linguistic tasks, but when he or she has grasped what he or she is being asked to do, he or she does it. A properly conducted sleep EEG should follow revealing electrical status epilepsia in sleep (ESES). Appropriate treatment should then ensue.

Sometimes psychological deficits manifest with surgical precision. I recall a 12-year-old boy who was unable to understand speech and had age appropriate reading and writing skills. In other children, inability to understand language extends to incomprehension of environmental sounds. There is frequently an accompanying behavioural disorder that seems greater than a reaction to a world that has become confusing.

Other epilepsies also carry this signature EEG. What is the relationship between LKS and, for example, rolandic epilepsy or the epileptic frontal and opercular syndrome? Classic LKS arises in a previously normal child. What are the taxonomic implications for a child with a pre-existing language disorder—and do they matter?

These and other issues are fully explored in this book, which the authors, after many years' experience and reflection, are uniquely qualified to write. They consider the recently proposed concept of the 'epilepsy-aphasia spectrum', in which conditions share involvement of the perisylvian networks of speech and language, which may be permanently affected. They explore the nature of this involvement. Does abnormal electrical activity directly damage circuitry or is some process affecting neuronal excitability and the primary pathology (or both in some malignant spiral)? They point out that the phenotype, especially with LKS of early onset, may mimic autistic spectrum disorder and address the relationship between autism and LKS.

They describe how management will involve not only the child neurologist but also professionals in the communication sciences, behavioural management and teachers of the deaf. Language as well as speech may be variably affected from one child to another, and management will have to be tailored accordingly.

They demonstrate how LKS can teach us much about the relationship between other epilepsies and cognitive function. We are fortunate that the authors' experience enables them to give a historical account of the development of our understanding of LKS, and also draw lessons from the pitfalls we have encountered along the way.

The reader will gain not only an understanding of LKS and related syndromes, but also a deeper appreciation of the relationship between epilepsy and related neuropsychological difficulties.

Richard Robinson
Emeritus Professor of Paediatric Neurology
Guys, Kings and St Thomas Hospital
London, UK

PREFACE

It was in the early 1970s that I first met a child who presented with loss of language comprehension, mutism and cognitive regression. He had only a few seizures, but severe epileptiform discharges on his EEG. He was thought to have an unusual kind of viral encephalitis until the unexpected course of the disorder, literature search, and discussion with colleagues prompted the recognition of similar cases in our community. We were faced with a mysterious combination of aphasia and epilepsy, without any evident cause, about which little had been written after the initial paper published by Landau and Kleffner in 1957. The prevailing hypothesis was that the epilepsy was an epiphenomenon of one or several different brain diseases, although the search for them remained elusive. During the same period, like many child neurologists around the world, we were busy in Lausanne trying to better identify the 'idiopathic focal epilepsies of childhood', a group of focal epilepsies without any identified structural lesion and a self-limited 'benign' course that seemed to occur quite frequently in otherwise typically developing children. While doing so, we became increasingly aware, like several others, of the many, but long unsuspected common features between rolandic epilepsy (or childhood epilepsy with centro-temporal spikes) and 'acquired epileptic aphasia' that unfortunately became known as Landau–Kleffner syndrome, an eponym that Landau and Kleffner themselves disapproved. The often remittent-relapsing course and, at times, spectacular remission of clinical and epileptiform EEG abnormalities (most prominent in sleep) with antiepileptic drugs or steroids clearly pointed to a direct role of the epileptic activity. Affected children exemplified the fact that an epilepsy can manifest with an acquired, insidious and puzzling disruption of language as well as other cognitive and behavioural functions. The latter can sometimes present like a developmental language disorder or an autistic spectrum disorder, whereas epileptic seizures can be rare or even absent. In short, epilepsy can no longer be regarded only as a paroxysmal disorder with various seizures types but can also present as a continuous slow progressive disorder with no evident paroxysmal features.

This prompted us to focus our research on longitudinal studies of children whose epilepsy was accompanied by a cognitive regression, developmental arrest or behavioural disruption. The aim was to try to disentangle a possible direct role of the epilepsy from all other factors that may affect cognitive function, and this in any epilepsy, regardless of type, cause or age at onset. This was a tedious, unspectacular approach, involving often single or only a few cases, each child being his or her own control. Such cases are often dismissed as anecdotal, but we thought, and still think, that their study is justified given the paucity of relevant data that emerge from many group studies and their tendency to disregard exceptional but informative cases. This led us to our first book titled *Cognitive and Behavioural Disorders of Epileptic Origin* (Deonna and Roulet-Perez 2005). Since then, several new tools in the domain of electrophysiology, functional imaging, genetics, neurometabolism and neuro-immunology became increasingly used in children with epilepsy, including Landau–Kleffner syndrome and rolandic epilepsy. They contributed to show that despite their many differences, these syndromes belonged to a continuum.

This diversity of the 'epilepsy-aphasia spectrum' is mirrored by that of the numerous medical and non-medical professionals who studied children at various points in the course of the disease, usually focusing on one selected aspect and published in a multitude of different periodicals or book chapters in the past 50 years or so.

About 10 years after my encounter with my first patient and involvement in this topic, I was fortunate to be joined by Eliane Roulet-Perez who became a life-long collaborator and my successor as the head of child neurology in Lausanne University Hospital. She became from the start an enthusiastic partner on all childhood epilepsy issues that we studied. She carried out pioneering studies of epilepsy with continuous spike-waves during sleep, on sign language in Landau–Kleffner syndrome, cognitive development of young children after successful epilepsy surgery and epilepsy in glucose transporter deficiency. This background and her fully active clinical and scientific involvement were decisive for me to dare to undertake the long-considered project to bring together the old and the new of the vast but scattered information on Landau–Kleffner syndrome and its continuum after my retirement. We both believe that the cognitive consequences of epilepsy are the most important aspect of childhood epilepsy in general and that the study of the children with epilepsies in the epilepsy-aphasia spectrum provides a helpful model for approaching many other epilepsies, including those with structural lesions.

It was also a last opportunity for me to bring to light forgotten and unpublished case histories and long-term follow-ups and describe the evolution of some older patients with Landau–Kleffner syndrome whose fate constitutes a now partly closed chapter in the history of this disorder. The dramatic loss of verbal comprehension and speech that has puzzled our forefathers in psychiatry and neurology has also allowed us to explore the history of ideas on many aspects of cognitive and social development of children and its disorders. It also allowed us to admire the adaptation of children to these extreme circumstances including the world of the deaf and the use of sign language.

There is a growing awareness that a full understanding of the consequences of brain disease on cognition and behaviour requires also an analysis 'at the first person' level. This subject-oriented approach is obviously difficult with children who either may not have enough insights or enough verbal understanding or ability to engage in a dialogue about their experience and emotions or even may have forgotten (or suppressed) memories of painful events. When possible, and with the help of their parents, we tried to give them a voice throughout this book and in the testimonies at the end, a dimension that cannot be found in short scientific papers.

Thierry Deonna
March, 2016

REFERENCE

Deonna T, Roulet-Perez E. *Cognitive and Behavioural Disorders of Epileptic Origin in Children*. Clinics in Developmental Medicine No. 168. London: Mac Keith Press, 2005.

ACKNOWLEDGEMENTS

Who, in our 'e-days', still supports the idea of writing a medical book, the more so on a complex and poorly understood topic in which new data accumulate constantly? A few colleagues and friends thought there was still room for such an endeavour and challenge, and their early encouragement was decisive: Jean Aicardi (now deceased), Peter Baxter, Claude Chevrie-Muller, Mary Coleman, Marie-Noelle Metz-Lutz, Isabelle Rapin and Patrick Van Bogaert. Our gratitude goes to all of them.

Most of the neuropsychological data on our patients were obtained by Claire Mayor-Dubois, the head neuropsychologist of our unit. Thanks also to her training in speech therapy and a great interest in language and Landau–Kleffner syndrome, we were able to investigate our patients in depth and follow them up over many years. Her contribution to several unpublished personal case reports is specifically mentioned throughout this book. We thank her for all her inestimable work and stimulating discussions during the preparation of this book.

We are indebted and thankful to Xavier De Tiège, Patrick Van Bogaert and Serge Goldman and their colleagues who wrote an important chapter on functional neuroimaging in the epilepsy-aphasia spectrum. We very much appreciate their willingness to contribute with their unique expertise in an otherwise personal book. They share with us the belief that the close integration of clinical and highly technical and sophisticated data is of paramount importance.

Several colleagues around the world whom we know personally or from their writings were kind enough to comment and go back to their own often old articles for a requested clarification or follow-up data: Claude Chevrie-Muller, Ine Cockerell, Alexander Datta, Peter Huppke, Mariko Kaga, Mary King, Sara Kivity, Christian Korff, Catherine Labasse, Peter Marien, Marie-Noelle Metz-Lutz, Juan Narbona, Geneviève Offermans, Costanza Pagano, Gunilla Rejnö-Habte-Selassié, Peter Ulldall, Patrick Van Bogaert and Paolo Veggiotti. Some of them and others, Prakash Kotagal, Sarah von Spickaz, Ulrich Stephani and Peter Uvebrandt, also provided us with the unpublished observations presented in Chapter 14. We are very grateful and indebted to them for the hard work they did to go back into their files.

Many of those mentioned above also read and made invaluable comments on the whole or selected chapters of our manuscript, as did Anne O'Hare, Richard Robinson, Anne-Claude Prélaz, Ingrid Scheffer and last but not least Anne-Lise Ziegler, an essential contributor in our initial projects. Many collaborators from our team and from the EEG and Neuroradiology of le Centre Hospitalier Universitaire Vaudois (CHUV), Lausanne who cannot be all named helped obtain invaluable data on our patients and we are grateful to them.

It is a great pleasure to also thank all the parents and children for their willingness to collaborate and accept investigations that they knew were not always for their direct benefit. This always makes a huge difference. Several patients were not children anymore, but adults accompanied at times by their elderly parents, when they accepted a late first or follow-up encounter and sometimes to be the subject of a special investigation.

We are indebted to CHUV, Lausanne and especially to Professor Pierre-François Leyvraz, the general director, for a grant that helped to support our project. We also thank Fabrice Weyermann for his very helpful local technical assistance. Finally, we would like to warmly thank our editors, Udoka Ohuonu and Ann-Marie Halligan, for their patience, encouragement and editorial guidance and our families and friends for their understanding when we were absorbed in our work.

TD and E R-P

1
INTRODUCTION

The idea that LKS is a rare condition that does not deserve a whole book has been gradually challenged over the years. Actually, language loss which is the hallmark of Landau-Kleffner syndrome (LKS) is only the most obvious and dramatic among a wide range of cognitive disturbances that can occur in the course of idiopathic focal epilepsies (IFE) of childhood, which are the most frequent childhood epilepsies. It has taken almost half a century to understand that LKS was due or closely related to a bioelectrical dysfunction of the brain, - ie. an epilepsy-even if it did not appear so at first glance. LKS has thus opened the way to the concept of "epilepsies with cognitive symptomatology" or "cognitive epilepsies", denoting those epilepsies that manifest mainly or exclusively in the cognitive or/ and behavioural sphere without (or only rare) seizures. (Deonna, 1993a; 1996; Deonna and Roulet, 2005).

LKS gradually emerged as a 'new' form of childhood aphasia following the publication of Landau and Kleffner in 1957 entitled 'Syndrome of acquired aphasia with convulsive disorder in children'. These authors reported six previously normal children who rapidly or more insidiously lost their language without any evident cause. However, they all had epileptic seizures except one and severe epileptiform abnormalities on their electroencephalogram (EEG). These disappeared after a few years and the aphasia recovered to various degrees. There was no other sign of brain dysfunction or evidence of a demonstrable acquired brain pathology. The language deficit involved mainly comprehension and was prolonged, unlike typical childhood aphasias due to focal brain lesions in language areas. Whereas antiepileptic drugs controlled the rather rare seizures, they seemed to have no effect on the language disorder or on the EEG, an observation that delayed the recognition of the direct role of the epilepsy. However, Landau and Kleffner already suggested that 'persistent convulsive discharge in brain tissue largely concerned with linguistic communication results in the functional ablation of these areas for normal linguistic behaviour'. A number of similar cases were subsequently recognized worldwide and assessed with new imaging techniques as they emerged. With rare exceptions, the latter never revealed a structural brain lesion. The eponym 'Landau–Kleffner syndrome' was introduced as an epilepsy syndrome equivalent to 'acquired epileptic aphasia' for the first time in the 1989 International League Against Epilepsy (ILAE) proposal for revised classification of epilepsies and epileptic syndromes. Over the years, the increasing recognition of new patients, follow-up of the early ones and an enlarged perspective on the age-variability, severity and role of the epilepsy have gradually led to the present view of LKS, which is summarized

TABLE 1.1
The early (1980–1990) and present (2015) views of Landau Kleffner syndrome

Early view (1980–1990)	Present view (2015)
Acute or insidious onset of aphasia (3–7y)	Also much younger, merging with developmental language disorder
Bitemporal FSW or spikes	Often CSWS in the active phase
Language deficit, mainly auditory agnosia	Also other speech and language deficits, other associated cognitive, behavioural and motor impairments
Chronic course, variable recovery	Mild forms with full recovery
Correlation aphasia and 'epileptic EEG' uncertain or dismissed as an epiphenomenon	Direct role of epilepsy on basis of pre-existing (genetically determined) abnormality of perisylvian networks
No lesions on brain imaging	Functional focal PET of (f)MRI abnormalities
Response to antiepileptic medication variable,	Steroids or ACTH very responsive and several AEDS helpful
Aetiology unknown and some cases with 'lesions' (see text)	LKS: Severe end of the IFE and EAS spectrum (rolandic epilepsy)

ACTH, adrenocorticotrophic hormone; AEDs, antiepileptic drugs; CSWS, continuous spike waves during slow sleep; EAS, epilepsy-aphasia spectrum; FSW, focal sharp waves; IFE, idiopathic focal epilepsies of childhood; PET, positron emission tomography

in Table 1.1. LKS is now considered to be at the severe end of a spectrum of epilepsy syndromes with neuropsychological deficits belonging to the idiopathic focal epilepsies of childhood (IFE), rolandic epilepsy being at its mild end (see Chapter 3 for further discussion). Now brought together under the broader label of epilepsy-aphasia spectrum (EAS), these epilepsies share an age-related, self-limited course, sleep activated interictal discharges (IED), response to similar medications and absence of a structural lesion. They are likely to be related to and linked together by a complex genetically determined alteration of maturation of the perisylvian networks supporting speech and language functions. Symptoms mainly consist in acquired, sometimes subtle language impairments. Other cognitive functions may also be affected when the focal epileptic activity shifts or spreads beyond the perisylvian region. Patients may thus present with executive deficits or a global intellectual, behavioral and even motor regression, that often correlate with the finding of intensely sleep activated diffuse and ample interictal epileptiform discharges (IEDs) on the EEG, called continuous spike waves during sleep (see chapter 3). The latter seem to sustainably modify the activity of more remote functionnally connected cortical areas such as the prefrontal regions via the thalamo-cortical circuitry (chapter 11).

Occasionnally, when an EAS syndrome starts very early in development, it can mimick a developmental language disorder or an autistic spectrum disorder (see chapter 6).

Beyond its status as an epilepsy syndrome, LKS has also helped clinicians understand that an acquired language disturbance in a child is not necessarily a sign of global cognitive regression or deafness, and it can have a neurophysiological rather than a psychological origin. Because of the affected cognitive functions and their consequences on the child's communication and intellectual development, the expertise of professionals outside the child neurology and epileptology fields is required, the management of the epilepsy being often only part of the story. LKS has, therefore, also captured the minds of specialists in communication sciences, speech pathology, neuropsychology and child development. It has also led to more fundamental questions. For instance, whether and how the different components of developing language can be selectively and temporarily disrupted and compensated for later on? How can a young human being cope with a prolonged loss of language while keeping otherwise preserved intellectual and emotional abilities and adapt without losing his or her essential self? What are the best ways to help the child to recover? If the child does not, how to maintain communication? Will he or she be able to learn a visual form of language, and if yes, how should it be taught? How did patients who recovered live the unique experience of being part of two different worlds, that of the 'deaf' and that of the hearing?

We believe that a historical review and a synthesis of the extensive but scattered research of the past 50 years on LKS and related epilepsy syndromes represent a fascinating journey into what is probably the most important aspect of childhood epilepsy, that is, its impact on developing higher cerebral functions. Many clinical and theoretical issues relating to LKS constitute an excellent introduction to this topic that has become a major preoccupation in childhood epilepsy and generates extensive research. The thinking about LKS proposed here can to a large extent be generalized to many epilepsies, including lesional epilepsies in which developmental stagnation, regression and various cognitive and behavioural impairments can occur beyond what is expected from the underlying aetiology and that propagate within one or both hemispheres and become activated by sleep.

Recounting the slow evolution of ideas, conceptual errors and late recognition of retrospectively obvious facts about LKS is a lesson of humility for all, a lesson that can apply to many other medical conditions. In this book we also report the tragic case histories and pay tribute to the early patients diagnosed with severe forms of LKS who we have met personally or read about in the literature. They were born when LKS was still unrecognized or diagnosed late and were badly managed. Some of these children have never spoken again and did not recover language comprehension either. It was difficult to find a place for them in schools, as they were not intellectually disabled or psychiatrically disturbed and were rarely accepted or at ease in schools for the deaf and the deaf community. In fact, they belonged to neither world. Such patients are now fortunately the exception, thanks to improved diagnosis, better drugs and better management. But so that the earlier patients might be forgotten by younger generations, we have given their stories a separate place at the end of the book.

2
THE HISTORY OF LANDAU–KLEFFNER SYNDROME

The Landau–Kleffner syndrome (LKS) represents a unique opportunity to look at early ideas about language and particularly its development and acquired deficits. It is often only when we are faced with a new or exceptional phenomenon that we start to think about what we normally take for granted. There is no reason to believe that LKS was a new condition that appeared at the mid-turn of the twentieth century. In other words, it certainly always existed, and descriptions of children who became mute for a long time or for the rest of their lives can be found in the medical or related literature. They must have intrigued the first psychiatrists, neurologists or other curious and compassionate men, who were willing to record their encounter with such an incomprehensible and tragic situation. The ways they tried to explain the cognitive disturbance of a patient, which we now would label as 'severe LKS', provides an insight into the history of ideas about complex brain function, and into the development of specific neuropsychiatric disciplines in the past hundred years. It is thus worth starting our journey as early as possible, looking at published cases whose description suggests a diagnosis of LKS, and see how they were interpreted before the advent of electroencephalography (EEG) in the early fifties.

The historical period before LKS was recognized
Table 2.1 shows the different diagnostic labels given by the emerging psychiatric and neurological fields for children with LKS before it was recognized, each with its own experience, bias and theoretical models.

THE ORIGINAL CASE
Probably, the first detailed description of a child that corresponds to LKS with verbal auditory agnosia (VAA) – inability to comprehend and repeat speech – (see Chapter 5) was published by Otto Pötzl (1877–1962) in a paper entitled '*Uber sensorische Aphasie im Kindesalter*' [Sensory Aphasia in Childhood]. A 7-year-old German child presented with acquired reversible sensory aphasia (half-year duration) and had 'episodic worsening of the aphasic disorder' The child was studied from January to November 1925 when he was back to normal in regular class. He expressed himself (in German) as such, 'I could not understand, because I did not hear you, but now I understand everything'. No

TABLE 2.1
Diagnostic labels given for Landau–Kleffner syndrome in emerging disciplines

Psychiatry: Dementia-aphasia

Psychoanalysis: Psychogenic mutism

Adult neurology: Word deafness and Wernicke's aphasia

Pediatric neurology: New form of childhood aphasia (different from childhood aphasias due to acquired
  focal brain damage)

Child neuropsychology: Acquired verbal auditory agnosia

epileptic seizures were reported, and this was 5 years before the invention of the EEG by Berger.

The description of the symptoms with the initial suspicion of deafness (ruled out by Pötzl with formal hearing tests), the rapid progressive course with fluctuations, the recovery over 6 months are fully consistent with a moderately severe and spontaneously remittent form of LKS.

Pötzl was a well-known Viennese psychiatrist and neurologist who at that time was a professor of psychiatry in Prague. He probably discussed this case at the Third Congress of the International Association of Logopedics and Phoniatrics, which was founded in 1924. Pötzl's introduction of his 26-page long article was to describe a so far unreported childhood sensory aphasia and to see how it differed from the already well-known (to neurologists) adult aphasias described by Wernicke and Liepman 30 years before: He discussed at length all existing data on acquired childhood aphasias and also included a discussion on the congenital word deafness. He was aware of the fluctuating symptoms that he had seen in adult chronic aphasias and that sensory aphasias could be epileptic phenomena. He even mentioned a case with the word deafness in a child with epilepsy that had worsened and in another one with 'petit-mal' seizures. Among possible aetiologies, he thought that an encephalitis or a conversion disorder were ruled out, and that ['the kind of disease involved must remain fully open']. Being uncertain about aetiology and without a specific hypothesis, Potzl realized that 'best observations of this kind' are in a 'borderland' and are likely to be seen by ear specialists or paediatricians'. He argued that they should be seen by neurologists to better understand the nature of their aphasia, and it was thanks to his colleague and friend Piffls that he had had this opportunity. The necessity of collaboration between different specialists, which are now considered very important, was by this time already acknowledged but subsequently lost with the increasing specialization and separation of disciplines.

LANGUAGE LOSS SEEN AS THE FIRST SIGN OR AN INTEGRAL PART OF HELLER'S DEMENTIA

In 1908, Heller wrote a seminal paper entitled '*Über Dementia infantilis*' (on infantile dementia) based on the observation of six children. These were previously typically developing and regressed between the age of 18 months–6 years to a 'state of idiocy', without any obvious precipitating illness, and they remained unchanged for years. In 1930, he reported having seen 28 similar patients. Rapin (1965) reviewed all published cases in the literature and concluded that it was not a homogeneous group. She stated that 'Some undoubtedly were psychotic or schizophrenic, others suffered from a number of diverse unrelated organic processes'. Epilepsy was not discussed as an important symptom or possible aetiology. Later, the children with acquired dementia and no identified aetiology were described as having 'childhood disintegrative disorder' (DSM-IV 1994) or 'childhood disintegrative psychosis'. These labels have been discarded in the (DSM-5 2013) and such children would now be merged into the broad category of 'autism spectrum disorders'. There is, however, controversy about the validity of this merger (Westphal et al. 2013) because the later age of regression, rapid onset, more global regression and presence of a prodromal phase of motor agitation and bizarre behaviours point to a distinct pathophysiology. 'Childhood disintegrative disorder' remains an umbrella term under which many different new diseases with a specific aetiology are increasingly discovered. It may, exceptionally, be the result of unrecognized and untreated epilepsy with continuous spike waves during sleep with prefrontal involvement (Roulet-Perez 1993; see Chapter 5).

Subsequently, the literature of the first part of the twentieth century until the 1960s suggests that the term 'dementia' was usually applied to children who lost language comprehension and expression without evident acute brain disease. However, description in some children indicated clearly that aphasia and not global cognitive regression was the main impairment (Jakab 1950; Lugaresi 1958; Koupernik et al. 1972).

A case described by Jakab (1950) in a paper entitled [Aphasia in Heller's dementia] is probably the most remarkable example of the erroneous concept of language loss as a main or integral part of dementia. The author, a neuropsychiatrist from Pécs University in Hungary, reported a 6-year-old girl followed for 14 months. She had transient language disturbances at 3 years 7 months and at 4 years 9 months; she had a sudden loss of language. She was said to have verbal deafness (*surdité verbale*) and was almost mute, able to utter only some vowels and repetitive syllables, part of her original language (Hungarian). She was unable to repeat words or phrases. She developed spontaneous gestures, and there is a detailed description of many intelligent non-verbal behaviours. The author ruled out 'hysteria', schizophrenia and oligophrenia, and the child had no symptoms suggesting an autism spectrum disorder.

Interestingly, the author made no comparison with the adult sensory aphasias and with deaf children using sign language. This suggests a lack of knowledge and of common thinking with the world of adult neurology or that of deaf children. Jakab, in her long discussion, classified her case as Heller's dementia, although she realized that ['as the only sign of dementia we find only the loss of speech and the inability to learn it anew'] (Jakab 1950). She commented that the girl had been left with 'an archaic form of thought' and had sustained a 'phylogenetic regression'. She seemed to consider that intelligence is always linked with verbal language. This is paradoxical because Jakab was obviously puzzled by the girl's clever adaptive behaviours. This remarkable case well illustrates the thinking of the early child neuropsychiatrists before psychonalysis invaded the field. Retrospectively, it is likely that this girl would have had LKS.

As late as 1958, Lugaresi reported a child whose 'fundamental trouble, is made of a total aphasia with conservation of the gestural language' (Lugaresi 1958). The translated title of the paper written in Italian was 'Aphasia in the infantile dementias' and the author in his English summary described 'the strict clinical relation of the case with Infantile dementia of Heller and the aparetic-aphasic phrenasthenia of De Sanctis'. He pointed out 'the exogenetic encephalopathic nature of the picture is evidenced by the presence of a serious epileptic dysrythmia'. Nothing in the clinical description however suggested that the child had a global cognitive regression. The EEG samples shown in the paper are typical of the frequent asynchronous focal sharp waves with generalized discharges seen in the active phases of LKS.

The same confusion between aphasia and dementia is also present in Kouperniks et al.'s paper (1969) entitled 'A case of Heller's dementia following sexual assault in a four-year-old girl'. Koupernik was a child psychiatrist with a biological and psychosocial approach and critical of psychoanalysis. Three years later, the same authors published a more detailed report and follow-up (Koupernik et al. 1972) on this child. This girl obviously lost speech, initially with paroxysmal episodes of anarthria, then had nocturnal attacks described as 'night terrors'. She was unable to understand language, had some spontaneous signing and was finally presented with a left focal motor status epilepticus. She had several EEGs that were initially inconclusive and only 4 years after she lost speech did the tracing show asymmetric spikes. The figure in their paper shows the typical focal sharp waves seen in LKS. At the age of 11 years, she had made no substantial progress. It is likely that she ultimately had a combination of a global aphasia with a cognitive and behavioural regression, the latter being neither the initial nor the most important symptom. The label 'Heller's dementia' was here hiding the main clinical features – that is, aphasia and epilepsy – and put the child in a 'waste basket' category, which was already well recognized as such during that time (Rapin 1965).

From the initial description by Landau and Kleffner to the present time
Landau and Kleffner (1957) reported that their six patients were suffering from 'a form of largely receptive aphasia'. They also describe expressive impairments in their case reports without further discussion (see Chapter 5). They mostly insisted on the differential diagnosis with peripheral deafness. (In fact, Franck Kleffner, the co-author of the paper, was the head of the Central Institute for the Deaf in St Louis, Missouri where he met some of these children.) The second historically most important and largest series of children was published 15 years later by Worster-Drought (1971), a speech pathologist, who had already written in 1930 about congenital word deafness. His paper was about 'an usual form of acquired aphasia'. He described his patients as having 'an acquired receptive aphasia as the main symptom' without further details. He suggested that the cause is 'a form of low-grade selective encephalitis, possibly of the autoimmune variety'. He did not consider epilepsy as a possible cause (as opposed to Landau's participants, which he knew about) because 'no epileptiform attack coincided with the onset of aphasia' (Worster-Drought 1971).

In 1977, Rapin, already then a leader among paediatric neurologists in the field of developmental language disorders (with one of the earliest comprehensive proposal of classification) and deafness, reported four ('possibly five') boys with 'acquired verbal auditory agnosia'. She distinguished her patients from adult Wernicke's aphasia, and made a clear anatomoclinical comparison with acquired 'pure word deafness' due to bilateral mid-temporal cortical lesions in adults (see Chapter 5). Remarkably, she described what Pötzl had already done 50 years before, but she did not mention his article. This seminal paper made pediatric neurologists aware that the combination of acquired verbal auditory agnosia and epilepsy without an evident aetiology was possibly a 'new' specific neurological syndrome.

It is almost by accident that the eponymic designation of LKS entered into the literature when Dugas et al. (1982) coined it in the title of a report on 12 children: ['Acquired childhood aphasia with epilepsy {Landau-Kleffner syndrome}'] in 1982. It was rapidly given authority in a paper of Dorothy Bishop, a renowned child linguist and neuropsychologist, the following year (Bishop 1985): She thought that LKS was an accepted medical designation (D Bishop, personal communication 2012) and focused her study on the influence of age at onset on outcome and comparison with acquired deafness. Her paper reinforced the idea that an acquired VAA was the defining clinical feature of LKS and led to the exclusion of other types of acquired speech and language deficits.

Deonna et al. (1977) reported six children with 'acquired aphasia in childhood with seizure disorder, a heterogeneous syndrome' and distinguished three clinical patterns: (1) those with rapid onset, frequent fluctuations of the aphasia and recovery; (2) those with worsening of the aphasia after repeated seizures or episodes of aphasia and (3) those with a progressive deficit in language comprehension (verbal auditory agnosia) and a variable degree of recovery with rare or no clinical seizures. These distinctions suggested the possibility of different aetiologies; some are directly related to the epilepsy, while others are probably not. Deonna et al. (1989) later became convinced, especially with the 10-year follow-up of their participants, and many others published since then that these different courses resulted from variations of a similar epileptic process and not from different diseases.

The search for aetiology and pathogenesis

There have been three lines of thinking on the aetiology and mechanism of LKS. First, a given brain pathology was at the origin of the aphasia and the epileptiform activity, the latter being only a 'by-product' of this pathology. Second, a structural lesion is responsible for the epilepsy that in turn caused the aphasia. Third the epilepsy itself is due to an intrinsic change of excitability in perisylvian circuits, causing the aphasia through short- and long-term effects on the language networks. Before the period when LKS became recognized as a non-lesional epilepsy belonging to the EAS spectrum, including rolandic epilepsy, clinicians were very eager to find a cause for this unexplained clinical picture that they sometimes attributed either the aphasia or the epilepsy (or both) to an incidental-imaging finding as illustrated by the cases below.

We are not aware of post-mortem studies of the brain in LKS, but in some instances, histology was examined from biopsies and surgical samples.

The same aetiology is responsible for the aphasia and the epilepsy

The slow fluctuating, but eventually the non-progressive course of aphasia and epilepsy, has naturally led to look first for a form of chronic but self-limited encephalitis.

Lou et al. (1977) reported on four children with acquired progressive and fluctuating aphasia with a slow protracted course. The outcome was variable from fairly good to poor (mainly 'auditory verbal' residual deficits). Intelligence was preserved in all children. All had seizures and severe focal, bilateral independent epileptiform EEG abnormalies that disappeared on follow-up in three out of the four patients where it was mentioned. The diagnosis of a subchronic encephalitis was based on the finding of a lymphocytic infiltration of the meninges in a left temporal lobe biopsy, performed in one participant only, because of an increased activity on a Technetium single photon emission tomography. In a 24-year-old man, the seizure types (atonic and myoclonic), EEG findings and clinical course during childhood were consistent with 'atypical benign partial epilepsy' (see Chapter 3). He had a fluctuating language deficit and made a good recovery with 'subnormal auditory memory' as the only sequelae. Another remarkable historical case of suspected focal encephalitis was treated with temporal lobectomy by the Montreal Rasmussen group (McKinney and McGreal 1974). This case, summarized in the following, was re-published with more details and a follow-up was made 14 years later by Cole (1988) entitled 'The Landau-Kleffner syndrome of acquired epileptic aphasia: unusual clinical outcome, surgical experience and absence of encephalitis' (see Fig 2.1). Note that Rasmussen had published on what became known as the 'Rasmussen encephalitis' in 1958.

Case study

A child was first admitted at the age of 5 for 'recurrent loss of hearing', probably from the age of 4. He later had progressive but clearly fluctuating receptive and expressive language difficulties with speech regression. He never had any seizures, but despite this, he underwent a left temporal lobectomy at the age of 7 to eradicate an epileptic focus: 'The EEG showed slow and sharp waves in the post-central region'. There was improvement, but the deficit recurred and the aphasia continued to fluctuate (Mckinney and McGreal 1974). In Cole's (1988) paper 14 years later, a post-operative follow-up of one more year was given, and the patient was later lost to follow-up. A brief neuropsychological description mentions 'a partial verbal auditory agnosia', and 'difficulty discriminating between similar sounding words'. The drawing of the resected left neocortical temporal area included Heschl's gyrus (primary auditory cortex), which was resected because of persistent per-operative epileptform activity after removal of the anterior 5 cm of the temporal lobe (Fig 2A in Cole et al 1988). Neuropathogical examination of the surgical specimen was described: 'The cytoarchitecure of the cortex and underlying white matter showed only mild subpial gliosis. There was no evidence of inflammation or loss of myelin. The hippocampus and ependyma were normal'. Cole et al. finally concluded that 'the syndrome has certain biological features that resemble the benign epilepsies of childhood and may be the result of the unusual localization of the epileptic abnormality (Cole et al 1988)' (see below).

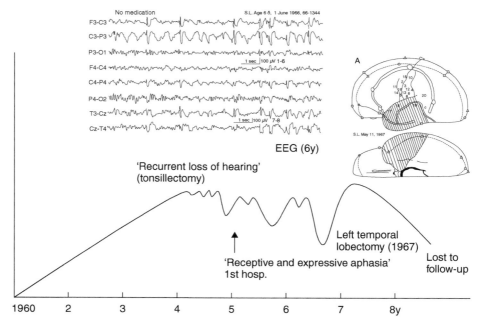

Fig. 2.1. A historical case of Landau-Kleffner syndrome treated by temporal lobectomy and follow-up. Top sections of figure reprinted from Cole et al. The Landau-Kleffner syndrome of acquired epileptic aphasia: understanding clinical outcome, surgical experience and absence of encephalitis Neurology 38:1 © 1988 American Academy of Neurology. Used with permission. Lower part of figure from adapted from McKinney and McGreal 1974.

A few additional biopsies of epileptogenic cortex have been obtained during multiple subpial transsection, a surgical procedure used in refractory focal epilepsies, performed in some children with severe and refractory LKS; see Chapter 12). Smith (1992) reported in an abstract 10 children 'a range of pathological abnormalities were found supporting the concept that LKS is a clinical syndrome of many possible aetiologies'. However, the final paper by the same team on multiple subpial transsection in LKS (Morrell et al. 1995) did not mention that topic again. Two large series after that (Irwin et al. 2001; Cross and Neville 2009) do not mention biopsies taken during the procedure: one of the co-authors of Irwin's series confirmed that no biopsies were taken (R Robinson, personal communication 2012).

Further discussions on the relation between the possible roles of inflammation and auto-immunity in LKS can be found in Chapters 8 and 12.

Acquired epileptic aphasia as a lesional epilepsy with different possible aetiologies
Several cases have been reported where a brain tumour, a focal encephalitis, cysticercosis or a focal brain malformation was found, or thought to be at the origin of the epilepsy, itself the cause of the aphasia (Otero et al. 1989; Perniola et al. 1993; Solomon 1993; Nass 1999a, b; Blum et al. 2007: Mikati 2009). Unfortunately, information on the type of language deficit

and its evolution in correlation with seizure frequency and EEG findings was often lacking, and together with the provided brain imaging and other laboratory findings, there was no strong evidence that the alleged brain pathology was indeed responsible for the symptomatology.

One of the four patients of the founding paper on LKS by Rapin et al. (1977) was found to have a vascular malformation on the angiogram. This was taken by many as an example of the many possible causes of the epilepsy in LKS. Eleven years later, however, Rapin and Allen (1988) published a courageous letter to the editor to the same journal stating that the patient with a left parietal angioma was restudied with brain MRI and that 'the reported anomaly was in all probability an overinterpretation of the findings'!

With this warning against incidental findings in mind, we must acknowledge that there are convincing historical cases of acquired epileptic aphasia due to a lesional focal epilepsy on record. At this stage, the question is if these should or should not be labelled as 'LKS' (see Chapter 3).

Two of them with pathological confirmation are summarized as follows:

Solomon et al. (1993) reported a boy aged 3 years and 6 months who 'developed partial-complex seizures with a right-sided motor activity occasionally secondary generalized with mild right Todd's paralysis at the age of 18 months'. Seizures were refractory and, at the age of 3, a 'rapid deterioration of language until occasional vocalizations occurred'. His EEG disclosed 'almost continuous bilateral generalized spikes, polyspikes, and spike-wave activity, worse during sleep' interically. Video-EEG monitoring revealed generalized tonic seizures with generalized ictal activity. A left mesio-temporal tumour involving the hippocampus and the parahippocampal region was found on brain MRI. Intracranial EEG monitoring through subdural strips under the temporal lobe and over the frontal lobe on the left side confirmed that the ictal activity started in the temporal electrodes before spreading to the frontal electrodes. After sub-total resection of the tumour—a low-grade astrocytoma—the seizures stopped within one month. After 6 months, language function was improved (no further information) and the EEG normalized.

A second case report of acquired epileptic aphasia with a definite brain pathology is a 30-year follow-up (Blum et al. 2007) of a patient from Gascon et al.'s (1973) initial small series (see below). The patient started with seizures at the age of 3 years and 6 months ('stomach-ache, glassed-eyed expression, and sucking movements of the mouth followed by sleep') and his speech deteriorated at the age of 4 years to become globally aphasic. A left temporal focus with bilateral spike and slow waves was found. At the age of 7 years, he became free of seizures but remained severely aphasic, albeit somewhat improved. Unexpectedly, seizures relapsed at the age of 20, and became increasingly refractory (mesio-temporal semiology with epigastric aura). A brain MRI at the age of 33 showed a left hippocampal T2 hyperintensity suggesting hippocampal sclerosis. He was operated at the age of 37, and histology revealed focal cortical dysplasia in the lateral temporal lobe and dyplastic neurons with gliosis in the hippocampus.

The authors gave a diagnosis of LKS because there was an epilepsy and acquired aphasia and 'the absence of a demonstrable lesion is not part of a clinical syndrome' (Solomon 1993). However, seizure types, seizure frequency and type of EEG abnormalities in Solomon's article did not correspond to those seen in LKS.

Huppke et al. (2005) found only one remarkable and convincing patient (a child) with an acquired epileptic aphasia who met the electro-clinical criteria of LKS but was found to have bilateral polymicogyria.

The child was followed from the age of 3 to 7 years with recurrent episodes of auditory agnosia. He had a typically developing language and speech development:

'At the age of 2 years and 6 months' dysarthria was first noted, but at that stage he still responded to requests. At age 3, he started to stutter and intermittently failed to respond to spoken words and other sounds. Over the following years he had periods where he could only communicate with his family using sign language and other periods where he was able to speak and understand words. These phases alternated every 2 to 3 weeks.

He was assessed at the age of 7: neurological examination revealed no signs of cortico-bulbar or cortico-spinal involvement. His EEG showed a few 'bilateral temporal spike discharges during the wake state. During slow-wave sleep, the epileptiform activity was found greater than 80% of the time in two recordings'. Brain MRI disclosed bilateral peri-sylvian polymicrogyria. The child responded well to sulthiame. According to the author who followed the patient until 2011 (Huppke, personal communication 2012), 'like in other cases with rolandic epilepsy, the EEG normalized during puberty and we stopped medication about 2 years ago. He still has minor speech problems but is otherwise doing very well'. The clinical symptoms, fluctuating course, EEG findings and final remission are similar to the typical non-lesional LKS with auditory agnosia, which it mimics perfectly also in its treatment response and ultimate remission.

Children with bilateral perisylvian polymicrogyria usually have developmental speech and language impairment as well as other impairments and often severe epilepsy (Kuzniecky et al. 1993). Dysplastic cortex may, however, be astonishingly functional and cause no or only mild epilepsy. However, this findings remains an exception in LKS because it has not been replicated in the now thousands of children with LKS who have undergone MRI (cf. Chapter 9 for further discussion).

Epileptic dyfunction as the main or only factor in LKS: a long road

There has been a 50-year discussion about the direct role of epilepsy in LKS. The view-points of clinicians who saw these children and studied them at different stages of the process and with different professional backgrounds are worth looking into, as often in history, ideas have gone back and forth. The main historical milestones are summarized in the Table 2.2.

The insight of Landau and Kleffner that 'persistent convulsive discharge in brain tissue largely concerned with linguistic communication results in functional ablation of these areas for normal linguistic behavior' (Landau and Kleffner 1957) was not pursued for a long time. The facts that some children never had any seizures, that they were not severe, and mainly that the aphasia was often chronic and not paroxysmal contributed to dismiss the epilepsy as the key player. In an influential paper based on 43 cases from the literature and two of their own, Holmes et al. (1981) proposed that 'epileptiform activity in this syndrome is an

TABLE 2.2
Role of epilepsy in Landau–Kleffner syndrome: history

Role of epilepsy in LKS: Clinical observation	First interpretation	Later findings
Aphasia not paroxysmal	Not epileptic	Fluctuations
No correlation between seizures and aphasia	Epilepsy not causal but epiphenomenon	Correlations between EEG abnormalites and aphasia exists, although not always time locked
Bilateral EEG abnormalities	Indicates diffuse brain disease	Bilateral independent EEG foci (mainly temporal) with sleep activation of discharges
No improvement of aphasia with antiepileptic drugs	Aphasia is not of epileptic origin	Worsening with sodium channel blockers (phenytoine and carbamazepine)More efficient AEDs and positive effect of steroids
Patients with focal brain lesions, focal encephalitis	Lesional epilepsy with aphasic symptoms	Rare lesional cases; LKS belongs to the rolandic epilepsy spectrum (EAS)

AED, antiepileptic drugs; EAS, epilepsy-aphasia spectrum

epiphenomenon reflecting underlying abnormalities of speech rather the cause of the aphasia'. This strong stance probably influenced many clinicians in rejecting or at least being very sceptical about a direct role of the epilepsy. It is even more interesting that Holmes later changed his mind and became a strong advocate of the role of interictal discharges in epileptic syndromes with language or other types of cognitive regression (Holmes and Lenck-Santini 2006; Chapman et al. 2015). The absence of a strict correlation between seizures, paroxysmal EEG abnormalities and evolution of the aphasia in many patients was indeed not suggestive of a direct role of the epilepsy. The often-diffuse epileptiform discharges or multiple foci on the EEG also suggested a rather extensive underlying brain pathology of unidentified cause. The observations that AEDS did not improve language and that the occurrence of a new seizure rarely had a worsening effect on language were for many the strongest arguments to dismiss an epileptic origin. It was later realized that the classical antiepileptic drugs used at that time (phenobarbital and phenytoïne) can have an aggravating effect on LKS, which was then unsuspected. Finally, even in those patients in which epileptic discharges were abolished with drugs such as diazepines, ethosuximide, sulthiame or steroids, there was rarely an immediate language recovery, similar to that expected in the ictal post-ictal deficit model. These classic ideas on epilepsy are well reflected in a paper entitled 'Language disorder, convulsive disorder and electroencephalographic abnormalities' published in 1973 in the by Gascon and three leading Harvard figures: the epileptologist Cesare Lombroso, who recognized rolandic epilepsy at the same time as Loiseau in France 1967 (see below); Harold Goodglass, a renowned neuropsychologist, and Norman Geschwind, the pioneering behavioural neurologist author of the twentieth-century classic model of the functional neuroanatomy of language gave 'critical suggestions' on the paper (Gascon et al 1973). They reported three children with an acquired language disorder and seizures with fluctuation of symptoms, speech arrest in one and bucco-linguo-facial deficits in another. The nature of the language deficit was not fully described, but severe comprehension difficulties were seen in all children. The EEG abnormalities were 'usually bilateral atypical spike-slow wave with posterior predominance (in patients 1 and 2)'. The authors considered all aetiological possibilities, including that the aphasia might be 'related in some unknown way to a convulsive disorder'. An argument against an epileptic aetiology was that one child who was given diazepam under EEG that suppressed the epileptiform discharges did not immediately regain speech. Surprisingly, the authors did not consider the fact that the child was already aphasic for 3 years and that this could play a role. At this time, a sleep EEG was not a routine and an increase of the waking abnormalities by sleep was not mentioned.

During the same period, and unrelated to the LKS issue, the Marseille school found almost continuous spike and waves during sleep without any obvious clinical correlate in children with epilepsy who presented with various cognitive-psychiatric impairments, but no severe seizures or signs of brain lesions (Patry et al. 1971). These were originally labelled 'subclinical status epilepticus induced by sleep in children' and became subsequently 'electrical status epilepticus during sleep' (ESES) (Tassinari et al. 2000), or 'continuous spike waves during slow sleep' (CSWS) (see Chapter 3).

A major sleep activation of the waking EEG abnormalities merging sometimes with CSWS was also recognized in some patients with rolandic epilepsy during the 1980s (Dalla Bernardina et al. 1978). *Sleep and Epilepsy* (1982) edited by Michel Billard, in which these pioneer studies were discussed, can be considered a landmark in the field. Since that time, and amply confirmed thereafter, came the crucial finding that children with LKS frequently have CSWS, especially in severe cases, or when a worsening of the aphasia is noted.

Morrell et al. (1995) performed pioneer electrophysiological studies in children with severe LKS and included electro-cortical recordings for presurgical work-up. The authors showed that a primary epileptic focus in the temporal region (either predominantly right or left sided) was driving the frequent and diffuse epileptiform discharges seen on the scalp EEG. This focus could be revealed when the latter was suppressed with barbiturates (see Chapter 9).

All these findings were taken together as evidence that LKS was a focal epilepsy without a structural lesion and that the focus triggered generalized epileptiform discharges, sometimes CSWS, through a mechanism of bilateral synchrony. The neuropsychological deficits were seen as related to the site of the focal epileptic process and its propagation. Later, these were also attributed to distant inhibitory effects of the epileptic activity beyond the propagation zone and to lack of memory consolidation provoked by CSWS (see Chapters 9 and 10).

The link between LKS and rolandic epilepsy in the older literature
The link between rolandic epilepsy and LKS took a surprisingly long time to be recognized and pursued, even though relevant features (clinical, EEG, and genetic) pertaining to this relationship were already observed in the historical cases.

These appear all the more significant as they were unbiased descriptions of patients with often a long follow-up that allowed the self-limited natural history of the disorder to be seen, excluding any unknown progressive brain disease.

LANDAU AND KLEFFNER'S ORIGINAL CASES

One of Landau and Kleffner's original cases (1957) already pointed to rolandic epilepsy. After a possible first seizure at the age of 4, a 9-year-old girl presented four brief tonic seizures 15 minutes apart on one evening. She recovered uneventfully and returned to school. During the next few weeks, however, she developed behavioural disturbances (withdrawal, temper tantrums, and nightmares) and she had progressive difficulty like 'stuttering' *leading to total absence of speech*. She had a single seizure relapse involving the right side of the face and body. At examination, she was a 'bright, friendly, cooperative child who seemed to enjoy the examination'. She responded to both oral and written commands and could give reliable answers to questions requiring 'yes' or 'no' answers. There was no spontaneous speech, but perseverative repetition of the syllable 'uni-ni-ni' on attempting to name pictures and objects. A month later, there was 'considerable improvement' and 6 months after onset, she had totally recovered. The first EEGs showed a left temporal focus of high voltage.

To conclude, this girl had an isolated acquired speech deficit with rapid full recovery, one single rolandic seizure during the acute phase and a high-voltage temporal focus on the EEG. On follow-up at the age of 32, she was fully normal (Mantovani and Landau 1980).

HARVARD TEAM IN THE GAME: NOT RECOGNIZING ONE'S OWN CHILDREN

The most surprising report is the already cited 1973 paper (Gascon et al. 1973). Despite the fact that the children they reported had episodes of 'speech arrest', simple focal motor seizures, a mild epilepsy course and temporal spikes, Lombroso did not make the connection with the epilepsy of the children he had himself reported in 1967 in a paper entitled Sylvian seizures and midtemporal spike foci in children. The latter turned out to be the same electro-clinical combination that Loiseau et al. had described in France the same year ['About a peculiar form of childhood epilepsy'] and that became universally recognized after the publication of an article by Beaussart (1972) in *Epilepsia* entitled 'Benign epilepsy in children with rolandic (centro-temporal) paroxysmal foci'.

THE FIRST PATIENT REPORTED WITH 'ACQUIRED VERBAL AUDITORY AGNOSIA' HAD A DAUGHTER WITH ROLANDIC EPILEPSY (RAPIN ET AL. 1977)

In this case (see case report with figure in Chapter 5, p.39), the fluctuations of the aphasia and of the EEG abnormalities with clusters of focal sharp waves, mainly in temporal location with shifting side preponderance and density with final disappearance and rare seizures (nocturnal) displayed on the figure in the paper are in keeping with an epilepsy belonging to the rolandic epilepsy spectrum. The patient was followed-up until adult age and made a full language recovery. Remarkably, his daughter has been diagnosed with rolandic epilepsy (I Rapin, personal communication. 2012).

A definite link between LKS and rolandic epilepsy: the late encounter
The concept that LKS was an epilepsy syndrome of its own and that VAA was an essential feature led to the disregarding of patients who started with a typical rolandic epilepsy and later became aphasic, those who had a speech or a language deficit different from VAA or those who had behavioural or additional cognitive impairments. In addition, the world of epileptology and that of educational and language sciences rarely met. On one side, epileptologists were in a fruitful phase of defining the different types of epilepsies and delineating epilepsy syndromes with the clearest possible boundaries. At this time, the concept of 'benign' epilepsies, meaning rare seizures and full remission occurring in otherwise typically developing children was dominant. 'Orthodox' clinicians therefore doubted that children with developmental or acquired cognitive and behavioural impairments could basically have the same type of epilepsy, and they tended to exclude them from their studies. As already discussed, it also took time to accept the fact that epilepsy can directly interfere with cognitive functions in a subtle, prolonged continuous way and is not only a succession of paroxysmal events. On the other side, specialists in speech pathology, child psychiatry, communication sciences and special education who met children with LKS often in a chronic, severe or late stage had rehabilitative or more fundamental scientific concerns and little information about the clinical context.

The first hint of a common pathophysiological background between LKS and rolandic epilepsy came from the growing recognition since 1982 that children with LKS had similar epileptic and EEG characteristics (Dulac et al. 1983; Cole et al. 1988; Deonna 1991). Cole, (1988) in his abstract stated that, 'this syndrome (Landau and Kleffner) has certain biological characteristics that resemble the benign epilepsies of childhood and may be the result of the unusual localization of the epileptic abnormality'. He was, to our knowledge, the first in North America to make the analogy with rolandic epilepsy, 20 years after benign childhood epilepsy was recognized (Lombroso 1967; Loiseau 1967). It took a bit longer to report children who started with a typical rolandic epilepsy but later presented with prolonged more or less severe reversible oromotor and/or expressive speech deficits. The EEG findings and fluctuating course were similar to many children with LKS except that the focal epileptic activity originated in the lower rolandic region (Roulet-Perez 1989; Deonna 1993; Shafrir and Prensky 1995; Kramer et al. 2001) (see Chapter 8). Later, large follow-up studies of rolandic epilepsy were published, in which a small proportion of children developed oromotor deficits, acquired auditory agnosia or more complex cognitive deficits (Fejerman et al. 2000; Saltik et al. 2005; Tovia et al. 2011). It is noteworthy that single cases of patients with rolandic epilepsy that evolved into LKS were reported with much doubt on the link between both (Yung et al. 2000; Berroya et al. 2004). Datta et al. (2013b) published the first longitudinally studied case of typical rolandic epilepsy evolving into LKS with rapid recovery documented through serial EEGs, EEG-source localization and functional MRI (see Chapter 8). The authors showed the successive localizations and bilateral propagation of the initial epileptic focus corresponding to the different clinical manifestations. Another compelling evidence came from patients with LKS in whom a history of rolandic seizures had not initially been recognized was forgotten (Deonna and Roulet-Perez 2005; and clinical vignette, case GA, Chapter 5) or occurred after the aphasia had recovered.

Table 2.3 summarizes the common features between LKS and rolandic epilepsy that have progressively been uncovered.

TABLE 2.3

Summary of common features between Landau–Kleffner syndrome and rolandic epilepsy

Clinical overlap

Patients with rolandic epilepsy evolving to LKS

LKS with prior unrecognized or later diagnosed with typical rolandic seizures

RE with prolonged oromotor and speech deficit

Common epilepsy and EEG characteristics

Rare seizures, final remission before/at adolescence

Focal sharp waves or spikes in the perisylvian area, unilateral or bilateral often asynchronous with changing predominance.

Activation by sleep (focal or diffuse, up to CSWS)

Normalization of EEG with age

Neuropsychological deficits

Speech and language deficits, including auditory processing, also in rolandic epilepsy (subtle and transient)

Written language acquisition problems in rolandic epilepsy

Genetic features

Rolandic epilepsy and LKS in same sibship

Parent and child with one or the other clinical phenotype

Same genetic mutations in rolandic epilepsy/AES spectrum (*GRIN2A*)

3
CLASSIFICATION ISSUES

Landau–Kleffner syndrome, epileptic encephalopathy with continous spike-and-wave during sleep and benign epilepsy with centro-temporal spikes: misunderstandings behind labels

Landau–Kleffner syndrome (LKS) has long been considered a rare and strange condition of uncertain status. For instance, in the 1974 edition of the classic by John Menkes, *Textbook of Child Neurology*, there were only a few lines written by Marcel Kinsbourne in the chapter on 'Disorders of mental development'. In the edition 20 years later, it had moved to the section on 'Non-convulsive status epilepticus' under the name 'LKS', also an arguable place.

The International League against Epilepsy (ILAE) mentions acquired epileptic aphasia together with LKS for the first time in the proposal for revised classification of epilepsies and epileptic syndromes in 1989. It appears in the category of 'Epilepsies and syndromes undetermined whether focal or generalized', under the subheading 'with both generalized and focal seizures'. This diverse list included neonatal seizures, severe myoclonic epilepsy of infancy, epilepsy with continuous spike waves during slow wave sleep (ECSWS) and acquired epileptic aphasia, with LKS given in brackets.

Landau–Kleffner syndrome

The eponym 'Landau–Kleffner syndrome' carried for a long time the implication that an obscure new underlying rare brain disease had to be found to explain the aphasia (see chapter 'In search of aetiologies'). This led to a fruitless search for brain lesions and obscured for a long time its obvious connection with rolandic epilepsy. In addition, the conviction that LKS should only refer to children with acquired verbal auditory agnosia (VAA) prevented many professionals from recognizing that children with other types of acquired speech and language deficits could belong to the same epilepsy syndrome.

The hallmarks of LKS are speech and language regression and sleep-activated focal epileptiform activity in the perisylvian region (See Chapter 1). Seizures are not mandatory. A certain amount of language must have developed before the onset of the disease, although this development may not have been normal. When a child presents with VAA or absent language from the outset (i.e. without regression) and epileptiform discharges suggesting LKS, it can be labelled as 'possible early LKS' (cf. Chapter 6). Unlike other authors, we do not restrict LKS to auditory or VAA, but include all subtypes of aphasias. These are not always easy to typify (see Chapter 5). Subtle language deficits as well as oromotor and speech disturbances of variable severity that can occur in the context of an active rolandic epilepsy are not labelled LKS, but included in the continuum called 'epilepsy–aphasia spectrum (EAS)', as defined below.

Individuals with a lesion are sometimes diagnosed as having LKS: it has been argued that this diganosis is clinical, consisting in an association of an acquired aphasia and an epilepsy. This argument, however, omits to take into account the seizure and electroencephalogram (EEG) characteristics that are essential and defining features of an electro-clinical syndrome (Berg et al. 2010; see also Chapter 2). Others are reported as 'symptomatic LKS'. We do not favour these designations and will restrict here the term LKS to children who have an acquired aphasia with the electro-clinical features of rolandic epilepsy and no demonstrable structural pathology to account for the epileptic activity. The rare cases (see Chapter 2) of speech and language regression related to lesional epilepsies originating in the perisylvian or mesio-temporal region usually have different electro-clinical features and will be referred to as 'acquired epileptic aphasia (AEA) with a structural lesion'.

Electrical status epilepticus in sleep (ESES), continuous slow wave discharges in slow wave sleep (CSWS) epilepsy with CSWS, and epileptic encephalopathy with CSWS

The use of the acronyms ESES, CSWS or ECSWS (for epilepsy or epileptic encephalopathy with CSWS) is still controversial and a source of confusion at many levels.

The first issue is whether CSWS and ESES are synonymous; the second is how frequent CSWS must be in order to be 'continuous'; the third is whether epilepsy with CSWS is an epilepsy syndrome and is distinct from LKS and whether the addition of the term 'encephalopathy' is justified; finally, where is the place of aetiology in epilepsy with CSWS?

(1) *ESES versus CSWS*: For the authors who participated in the initial recognition of this EEG pattern, the first 'E' of ESCWS (Cantalupo et al. 2013) has been changed from electrical to encephalopathy, thus 'encephalopathy with status epilepticus during sleep'. Tassinari argues that the term 'status epilepticus' has the advantage over CSWS to refer to an electro-clinical condition and not only to an EEG pattern. In our opinion, however, CSWS is the preferred term because status epilepticus means that there is electro-clinical concordance, with the implication that cessation of the epileptic activity (when not too prolonged) is followed by rapid recovery, which is not the case here. In addition, status epilepticus does not stop spontaneously on awakening from starting again night after night when falling asleep as CSWS does. Another argument given by Tassinari's group in favour of the term ESES is that this term is more flexible than CSWS regarding the morphology (spike waves vs. spikes and diffuse vs. focal) and the continuity of discharges (almost continuous vs. continuous) required for the diagnosis (Cantalupo et al. 2013). This is true, but the use of ESES does not escape the need to define the inclusion criteria that are indispensable for both the clinician and the researcher.

(2) This leads to the second issue: What is meant by 'continuous' in CSWS? The initially proposed spike-wave index (SWI) for CSWS was defined as a spike-wave activity occupying 85% or more of slow wave sleep. The 85% threshold was an arbitrary figure. It was followed with unflinching devotion until it became obvious that in some

cases, the quantity of nocturnal discharges varied both overnight and between nights as well as over longer periods in the same child. The SWI also varies between children with similar neuropsychological deficits. This stringency resulted in the exclusion from studies of children having cognitive impairments as important as those found in 'typical' CSWS but not meeting the quantitative EEG criterion. Note that the ILAE classification proposals (1989) did not define any threshold SWI. Other sources of disagreement on CSWS criteria (Scheltens-de Boer 2009; Sánchez-Fernández 2012a) include how the SWI is calculated and morphological and distribution aspects of the spikes (e.g. spikes vs. spike waves and focal or bilateral focal vs. diffuse discharges). This complexity has resulted in the increasing use of various sleep-activation grading scales. One suggestion was that mild activation was defined by a SWI of 10%–50% of non-rapid eye movement (NREM) sleep, and strong activation by an SWI of 50%–85%, whereas CSWS was reserved for a SWI of 85%. Although the strict use of the 85% SWI has been widely adopted, a broader range of quantification of the SWI has clinical and scientific utility; for example, Losito et al.'s (2015) paper is a study that applies this kind of scale. We fully endorse the use of a graded scale of SWI and the application of other methodological guidelines that aim at unifying the way we look at CSWS (Scheltens-deBoer et al. 2009).

(3) Epilepsy with CSWS was classified by the ILAE in 1989 as an epilepsy syndrome in the category 'undetermined whether focal or generalized' and was differentiated from AEA (which was considered equivalent to LKS). The word 'encephalopathy' was added later in the ILAE report (Engel 2006; Berg et al. 2010). The concept of 'epileptic encephalopathy' can be applied to any epilepsy in which 'the epileptic activity itself may contribute to severe cognitive and behavioural impairments above and beyond what might be expected from the underlying pathology alone' (Berg et al. 2010). One can hence wonder here why it has been added to the label of only this specific epilepsy syndrome, whereas it does apply to many other syndromes, for example epilepsy with myoclonic atonic seizures. Another issue raised by the term 'encephalopathy is that it implies that the mental state is diffusely altered (level of consciousness, cognitive functions and emotional state), which is not always the case in ECSWS, where neuropsychological dysfunctions may be more specific and mild. In our opinion, a term like "focal epilepsy with neuropsychological deficits and CSWS" would be preferable and can be further specified when necessary. Neuropsychological patterns found in ECSWS like the "acquired epileptic frontal syndrome" are discussed in chapter 8. Here, the acronym ECSWS will designate the syndrome of epilepsy or epileptic encephalopathy with CSWS, whereas CSWS alone refers to the EEG pattern.

(4) ECSWS is an epilepsy syndrome in the same way as the well-recognized West and Lennox–Gastaut syndromes. It occurs both with and without a structural abnormality. A range of cerebral lesions can be associated with CSWS, including focal and bilateral polymicrogyria, perinatal cerebral infarction, shunted and non-shunted hydrocephalus and thalamic lesions. In several studies, children with ECSWS of different aetiology have been combined, rendering the interpretation of the effectiveness of cognitive

outcome treatments difficult. The electrical pattern of CSWS may also occur in LKS and leads to syndromic confusion. In this book, ECSWS will designate the epilepsy syndrome as that occurring in a non-lesional setting unless otherwise specified.

Idiopathic focal epilepsies of childhood

'Idiopathic focal epilepsies (IFE)' is a generic term used for a group of non-lesional focal epilepsies of childhood, the most common of which is rolandic epilepsy. The term 'idiopathic' is synonymous with 'intrinsic' or 'primary' and means that there is no cause other than a presumed genetic predisposition. Idiopathic is not completely overlapping with "non-lesional": the latter refers to what can be seen at a structural level and is of course a matter of scale and technical refinement. It is well known that some epilepsies considered as non-lesional even with good MRI techniques reveal at the end to be related to mild structural changes at pathology. Frontiers between "lesional" or "structural" and "functional" changes become increasingly blurred as imaging technology improves and can be of course a matter of debate. In this book, we will consider "soft-wired" dynamic changes at cellular or sub-cellular level like synapses, cytoplasmic transport systems or ion-channels which are likely substrates of "idiopathic" epilepsies as "functional" and not "structural". The term "non-lesional" is used here in a broader sense, meaning that an anatomical substrate has not been found, with the limits of the used or commonly available technique. In some instances, the term 'genetic' has replaced idiopathic where there is clinical or molecular genetic evidence of causation. In other cases where the aetiology is not known, the term 'unknown' is suggested (Berg et al. 2010; see also Chapter 9 on genetics). IFE includes syndromes such as early-onset benign occipital epilepsy, now called 'Panayiotopoulos syndrome', and late-onset childhood occipital epilepsy, called 'Gastaut syndrome'. These are sometimes grouped as 'benign occipital epilepsies of childhood'. A few less well-defined and rarer focal epilepsies with focal spikes or sharp waves in regions other than the centro-temporal regions are also recognized (Vigevano et al. 2013). It does not include other genetic, dominantly inherited, focal epilepsies starting in infancy or childhood–adolescence such as self-limited (former benign) familial infantile epilepsy, familial frontal, temporal or multifocal epilepsies (Vigevano et al. 2013). In this book, the label IFE will be used because classification issues about the use of the term 'idiopathic' in focal epilepsies are not yet settled.

Rolandic epilepsy, formerly 'benign' epilepsy with centrotemporal spikes

In the former label of the syndrome 'benign partial epilepsy of childhood', later renamed 'benign epilepsy with centrotemporal spikes' (BECTS), 'benign childhood epilepsy with rolandic spikes (BCERS)' or 'benign rolandic epilepsy' (BRE), the term 'benign' is a source of misunderstanding. Although benign refers to seizure outcome, it also implicitly means that the children are neurologically and cognitively normal and remain so during the course of the epilepsy. Consequently, many children with developmental delay before the onset of seizure or with acquired cognitive or behavioural disturbances were not considered as having this syndrome, and hence this was not studied for a long time. In the new classification proposal from the ILAE, the term benign has been deleted and replaced by 'self-limited', and the syndrome is now renamed as 'childhood epilepsy with centro-temporal spikes' (CECTS) (refer to Epilepsy Diagnostics Manual of the ILAE at www.epilepsydiagnosis.org).

Rolandic epilepsy as the prototype of idiopathic focal epilepsy

In this book, we have elected to use 'rolandic epilepsy' as a synonym for CECTS. It is commonly used in the literature with the advantage of being shorter, and it refers to the neuro-anatomy, the cortex adjacent to the central (rolandic) sulcus where the seizures originate – rather than to the EEG hallmark. Moreover, the interictal discharge is often a focal sharp wave rather than a spike and its location is not always strictly centro-temporal. Rolandic seizures, previously called 'sylvian' seizures, refer to their onset in the lower rolandic region with hemifacial sensorimotor and phaynrygeal seizures.

Seizures with rolandic semiology can also have a structural origin, but here rolandic epilepsy will be restricted to non-lesional 'idiopathic' epilepsy.

When does rolandic epilepsy become 'atypical'?

The adjective 'atypical' attached to rolandic epilepsy first appeared in the literature following a paper entitled 'Atypical benign partial epilepsy of childhood' (ABPE) published in 1982 by Aicardi and Chevrie. They reported four children with rolandic epilepsy who, in addition to focal motor seizures, had absence, myoclonic and atonic seizures. Their EEG showed focal paroxysmal epileptiform activity on the waking record that evolved into diffuse, almost continuous, slow spike waves during sleep. This clinical and EEG picture resembled the ominous syndrome of epilepsy with myoclonic atonic seizures, previously called 'Doose syndrome', and Lennox–Gastaut syndrome with which it was sometimes confused. However, after a stormy epilepsy course, the seizures fully remitted as did the EEG abnormalities and, initially, the children were thought to remain developmentally normal. It was later recognized, however, (J Aicardi, personal communication 1986) that mild cognitive deficits could occur. Later studies actually showed that these children often had classic CSWS with significant cognitive impairment during the active phase even if the ultimate outcome was favourable (Hahn et al. 2001).

Nevertheless, the term 'ABPE' remains in use, but the recently issued 'Diagnostic Manual' of the epilepsies (www.epilepsydiagnosis.org) replaced it with 'atypical childhood epilepsy with centro-temporal spikes' (ACECTS). In ABPE, however, the spikes may not be strictly centro-temporal, but rather centro-parietal, parietal or closer to the vertex (de Tiège et al. 2013).

In addition to ABPE, confusion arises because the term 'atypical' is also used to qualify rolandic epilepsy with unusual seizure characteristics (early onset, long duration or high frequency of seizures and additional seizure types such as negative myoclonus) or/and unusual EEG features (multifocal spikes, intermittent slow waves, burst of generalized spike waves and major activation of interictal focal activity merging into diffuse CSWS) that can predict unfavourable neuropsychological outcome (Massa et al. 2001; Saltik 2005; Fejerman 2009).

The adjective 'atypical' is also used to qualify the evolution of rolandic epilepsy when it becomes complicated by the occurrence of severe neuropsychological deficits and the finding of CSWS on the EEG (Fejerman 2009). This includes ABPE, LKS and ECSWS. In the *Handbook of Clinical Neurology* (2013, pp. 636-640), Van Bogaert states that 'there is now agreement to speak about "atypical rolandic epilepsy" when severe neuropsychological impairment that may become persistent occur in a child with BECTS in association with CSWS' an opinion with which we do not quite concur.

Thus, 'atypical rolandic epilepsy' remains, for all the above cited reasons, an ambiguous term and when it is used, authors should specify precisely what they mean. This leads to the necessity of finding better concepts that include rolandic epilepsy with a complicated course, such as the 'epilepsy-aphasia spectrum' discussed below. In this book, for the sake of clarity, we will keep the original label of ABPE when referring to this particular syndromic form of rolandic epilepsy, and atypical rolandic epilepsy will be used in its broader sense of an unusual course of rolandic epilepsy at the epilepsy or/and cognitive level.

Panayiotopoulos syndrome as a cousin of rolandic epilepsy

Panayiotopoulos syndrome (1999) manifests as infrequent, sometimes a single, nocturnal seizure in a child of younger age (2 to 4 years) than rolandic epilepsy. Seizures usually start with autonomic manifestations such as vomiting, pallor, sweating or pupillary changes (unilateral mydriasis), followed by alteration of awareness and eye and head deviation that can evolve into a unilateral or bilateral convulsion. Seizures are often prolonged evolving to status epilepticus, and they are mistaken for an acute encephalopathy because of the autonomic features. As opposed to rolandic epilepsy with a centrotemporal focus, there is more variability in the location of the epileptic foci in Panayiotopoulos syndrome, although there is an occipital preponderance. Frontal spikes that represent a secondary activation from the occipital focus can also be found (Leal et al. 2008) as well as generalized discharges, with or without associated focal discharges. Interictal focal or generalized discharges are activated by sleep as in rolandic epilepsy. EEG features often change over time, and repeated recordings can remain normal. In 20% of affected children Panayiotopoulos syndrome evolves into rolandic epilepsy with an anterior shift in the location of the main EEG focus from the occipital to the centro-temporal region. This overlap between syndromes has been referred to by some authors as the 'benign childhood seizure susceptibility syndrome' (Caraballo et al. 2011; Sánchez Fernández and Loddenkemper 2012).

There is no evidence that children with Panayiotopoulos syndrome have acquired oral or written language impairments such as those seen in rolandic epilepsy. Neuropsychological studies of Panayiotopoulos syndrome (De Rose et al. 2010; Bedoin et al. 2012; Lopes et al. 2014) reveal rare, subtle and variable disturbances, especially in visuospatial attention (Bedoin et al. 2012). One has to expect that potential deficits will be more difficult to demonstrate in Panayiotopoulos syndrome given the younger age of the patients and the more variable, often less sustained, interictal epileptiform discharges.

In this book, there will be no further discussion of Panayiotopoulos syndrome and other rare IFE syndromes, even though similar concepts regarding correlations between the

TABLE 3.1
The epilepsy-aphasia spectrum: a spectum at multiple levels

---

(1) *Epilepsy syndrome spectrum*:
No seizures to refractory seizures
Mild sleep activation of unilateral CTS to diffuse CSWS
Rolandic epilepsy, atypical benign focal epilepsy, acquired epileptic opercular syndrome, LKS and ECSWS

(2) *Spectrum of language and cognitive deficits*:
Developmental age spectrum – Developmental language disability/acquired aphasia
Localization spectrum – Anterior/posterior model (from 'sound to meaning' and 'sound to action' in the dual-stream model)
Neuropsychological spectrum – Specific speech/language skills versus global cognitive deficit with behavioural disorders. Oral versus written language deficit. Different subtypes of aphasia and underlying cognitive deficits

(3) *Phenotypic spectrum within families*:
Various developmental language and cognitive disorders in parents or siblings with/without seizures or focal epileptiform abnormalities (CTS). Same or different EAS syndromes in one family.

CTS, centrotemporal spikes; CSWS, continuous spike waves during slow sleep; ECSWS, epilepsy with continuous spike waves during sleep; EAS, epilepsy-aphasia spectrum

neuropsychological findings and the location, propagation and activation of the focal epileptic activity during sleep may apply (see Table 3.1 and comments).

The epilepsy-aphasia spectrum: a spectrum at multiple levels

The word 'spectrum' refers to either 'a range of values of a quantity' or 'set of related quantities' (as in physics) or to 'a broad sequence or range of related qualities, ideas or activities'. Both definitions can apply to the different facets of the EAS, as discussed below.

The EAS is a concept coined by Ingrid Scheffer in the context of understanding the childhood epilepsy syndromes, and is detailed in her group's work on the clinical genetics of these disorders (Vears et al. 2012; Carvill et al. 2013; Tsai et al. 2013; Turner et al. 2015a, b; see Chapter 9). The term 'aphasia' emphasizes that language deficits are a hallmark of these focal epilepsies of most likely genetic origin that predominantly involve the perisylvian regions. The EAS comprises rolandic epilepsy at the mild end. Then comes a broader less well-defined group named 'intermediate epilepsy-aphasia disorders (IEAD)' that refers to patients with mainly speech and language deficits and sleep-activated interictal discharges that do not meet the criteria for CSWS, either quantitatively (SWI index) or qualitatively (lateralized vs. diffuse discharges). The severe end includes the acquired epileptiform opercular syndrome (AEOS; see Chapter 9), LKS and non-lesional ECSWS.

Besides the sleep activation and epilepsy syndrome spectrum, the term spectrum can also apply to language and other cognitive dimensions. Recently, the authors of the EAS concept emphasised that: 'despite the use of aphasia in the term EAS, many patients do not experience complete loss of language and this word is used to denote a range of speech and language disorders' (Turner et al. 2015b). These may be considered from different perspectives, which in turn represent a spectrum:

(1) *The developmental age spectrum*: This refers to children with very early onset aphasia who are indistinguishable from those with a developmental speech and language disorder at one end and to older children with later onset and clearly acquired aphasia at the other.

(2) *The localization spectrum*: This refers to the posterior versus anterior location in the speech and language network, grossly corresponding with its receptive versus expressive dimension (see Chapter 4). At one end of this spectrum, children present with auditory or VAA, and at the other end are those with oromotor and speech deficits.

(3) *The neuropsychological spectrum*: At one end, one can find specific and isolated deficits, for example, regression in oromotor or in graphomotor skills and, at the other, global cognitive regression and severe behavioural disorders. Some children may have behavioural and social impairments akin to those seen in autism spectrum disorder. Within one complex domain, for instance speech and language, one can also analyse further dimensions such as the different affected linguistic components (e.g. articulation, phonological awareness and production and pragmatics) or modalities (oral vs. written language).

Finally, one can also consider the spectrum of phenotypes observed within a family: this refers to the findings that parents or siblings of affected children may also have various developmental speech and language and/or cognitive impairments with focal epilepsy or focal epileptiform discharges, such as centrotemporal spikes without seizures. Of interest is that the same or different EAS syndromes can be found in one family. Mutations in *GRIN2A* have been identified in 9%–20% of probands with EAS syndromes (see Chapter 9). In this book, the term EAS will be used with this multilevel spectrum perspective in mind (Table 3.1).

4
SPEECH PERCEPTION AND BRAIN ORGANIZATION OF LANGUAGE: RELEVANT FEATURES FOR LANDAU–KLEFFNER SYNDROME AND THE EPILEPSY-APHASIA SPECTRUM

Before describing the various speech and language impairments that have been reported in clinical studies of children with Landau–Kleffner syndrome (LKS) and the wider spectrum of EAS, it is worth summarizing some fundamental physiological facts about auditory and language perception as it pertains to oral language perception and comprehension. It may explain some unusual and sometimes isolated deficits or on the contrary, preserved language features seen in these epilepsy syndromes.

Acoustic features of speech and comprehension of connected discourse
The final aim of oral communication, probably unique to humans, is not only the understanding of short message about objects, facts, actions, direction or basic emotions but also the exchange of information and thought about the world in a larger sense, beyond the here and now. The successful enfolding of this process results from complex operations. These are depicted by Dorothy Bishop in her book *Uncommon Understanding: Development and Disorders of Language Comprehension in Children* (1997). A model of the different steps of speech processing from transforming a sound wave into meaning is shown with the example of a short sentence: 'The fish is on the table' (Fig 4.1).

In the original legend of the figure, Bishop states that 'in this model, comprehension is depicted as a purely "bottom-up process", with incoming information being subject to successive transformations in sequential order. As we shall see, this is a gross oversimplification' (Bishop 1997, p.3). 'Top-down processing', meaning that the listener's prior knowledge of the language, context and expectations, also strongly influences interpretation of the perceptual input at its different stages. This is particularly relevant to children with LKS (see subsequent text).

A *phone* is defined as the smallest identifiable sound unit found in a stream of speech, one of the many possible sounds of languages in the world - the domain known as phonetics. A *phoneme* is defined as a contrasting unit in the sound system of a given language, a

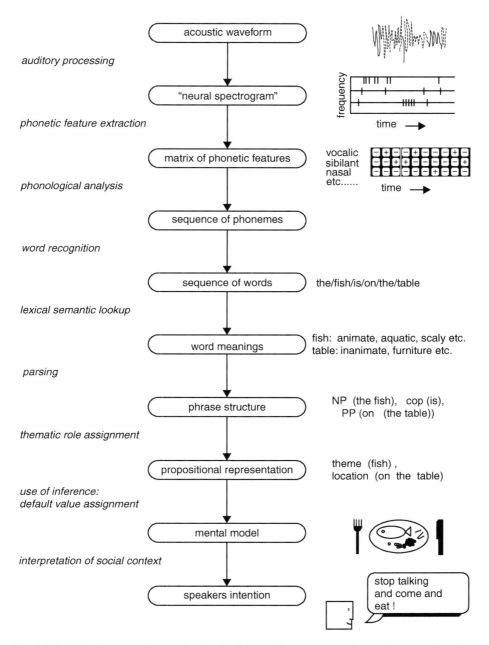

Fig. 4.1. Model of stages of proceesing involved in transforming a sound wave into meaning when comprehending the utterance: 'The fish is on the table'. (Reprinted from Bishop DVM, *Uncommon Understanding: Development and Disorders of Language Comprehension in Children*, Psychology Press, Hove, UK with permission from Taylor & Francis Group © 1997.)

minimal unit that distinguishes between meaning of words. (For instance, the sounds *b* and *p* are acoustically distinct phones in a neutral environment, but the phonemes /b/ in bark versus /p/ in park are part of English but not of Arabic phonology.) This is the domain known as phonology. A *syllable* is a unit of organization for a sequence of phonemes, often composed of a vowel with an initial and/or terminal consonant. For example, the word *meter* is composed of 2 syllables, *me-ter*.

Recent electrophysiological studies indicate that there are distinct neuronal populations with different intrinsic properties for processing the various attributes of sounds (low frequency/high freqency and short/long duration) (Tankus 2012). Some react to the constant changes that occur over the longer period (seconds) that are necessary for the understanding of connected speech. At the level of the word and more so at the level of a whole sentence (Fig 4.2), verbal understanding depends thus on the perception of complex acoustic pieces

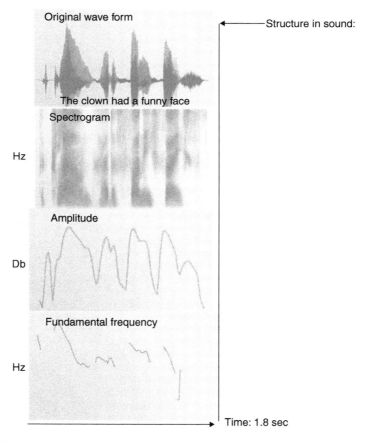

Fig. 4.2. Structure in sound in a sentence. (From Scott et al., A little more conversation, a little less action – candidate roles for the motor cortex in speech perception, *Nat. Rev. Neurosci.*, 10 (4), 295–302, 2009. Reprinted with permission from Macmillan Publishers Ltd.)

of information that propagate at variable speeds (featural information, i.e. rapid succession of consonants such as 'ts': 20–50 ms; syllabic information:150–300 ms; intonation level information: 500–1500 ms).

This means that the various acoustic components involved in a given message reach the brain at different time points, called 'multitime resolution analysis'. The sound frequency and loudness also vary a lot, depending, for instance, on the pronounced vowel in a syllable starting with a same consonant (see Fig 4.3) and are different across languages.

Figure 4.2 adapted from Scott et al. (2009) illustrates the various acoustic parameters (overall frequency, amplitude and fundamental frequencies) and their rapid changes that take place at different times through the production of a sentence: 'The clown had a funny face', which lasts 1.8 seconds.

In addition, there is a relative 'superiority' of the capacity of each hemisphere in the detection of different phonetic features, for instance, voiced – that is, using the vocal cords – consonants, as *b* or *d*, as opposed to voiceless – that is, not using the vocal cords – consonants, as *p* or *t*, are better proccessed by the right hemisphere (Bedoin et al. 2010).

Speech–sound perception (ability to differentiate between closely related phonemes) and speech recognition (meaning of word) can be affected separately (double dissociation) in pathological conditions.

This indicates that there are different possible routes to word recognition, one that bypasses the level of phonemic discrimination (= serial model) and goes directly from syllables to word (= parallel model). For a word to be directly recognized through this latter route, it must already belong to the child's vocabulary (top-down). See Figure 4.4.

LEVEL OF PERCEPTION DEFICIT IN VERBAL AUDITORY AGNOSIA

Auditory agnosia is defined as a deficit of recognizing sounds despite adequate hearing. It can be used in a broad sense of an incapacity to recognize speech and non-speech sounds and in a narrow sense – favoured by neuropsychologists and the authors of this book – of incapacity to recognize non-verbal sounds only.

Verbal auditory agnosia (VAA) (synonymous with auditory verbal agnosia or word deafness) denotes a selective impairment in speech–sound recognition. Auditory and verbal

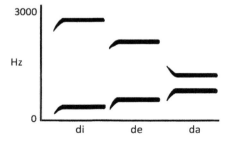

Fig. 4.3. Idealized spectrograms for three syllables. Spectrograms for three syllables di-da de da. (Adapted from Lieberman 1957)

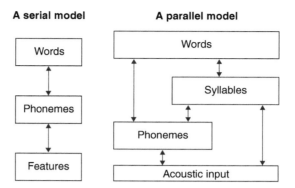

Fig. 4.4. Serial versus parallel models of speech recognition. (From Hickok, 2009.)

auditory agnosia can occur together – that is, global auditory agnosia – mainly in the acute period of cerebral lesions or of LKS.

There is a recurrent debate whether the deficit in recognizing words in VAA is due to altered perception of acoustic features of speech or due to a higher order deficit in phonological discrimination. The fact that non-verbal sounds, which can be complex to identify (inanimate versus animate, sounds of nature, human objects sounds etc.), are recognized, while decoding of phonemes or words is not possible has been taken to mean that a specific deficit in phonological discrimination is the problem (Korkman 1998). However, the recognition of meaning of sounds to be identified probably depends as much on the auditory characteristics of the non-verbal sounds to be identified as on word/non-word differences.

Functional neuroanatomy of language: a new model
Modern views on functional neuroanatomy of language have changed our classical concepts on language networks based on clinical-pathological observations. In the past 20 years, increasingly sophisticated functional brain imaging tools and language paradigms have brought a revolution in the neuroscientists' understanding of language processing (Poeppel et al. 2004). In the words of these authors

> The definition of and restriction to the few brain regions comprising the classical model dramatically underestimates the number and distribution of brain regions now known to play a critical role in language comprehension and production. Not just the role of the right (non-dominant) hemisphere has failed to be appreciated, but other left lateralized extrasylvian regions such as the middle temporal gyrus are now known to be essential, as is the involvement of subcortical areas.

The dichotomy between reception (language comprehension) and production (speech), and the stringent left-sided dominance for language do not hold true anymore, or for gross aspects of language processing only. Hickok (2009, 2012) have proposed a dual-stream model of speech processing: the ventral stream processes speech signals for word comprehension, and the dorsal stream maps acoustic speech signals to frontal and parietal articulatory networks. The ventral stream ('from sound to meaning') is largely bilaterally organized, but with 'important computational differences between the left and right hemisphere systems (Hickok and Poeppel 2007)'. According to the authors, It processes auditory information as follows:

> The earliest stage of cortical speech processing involves some form of spectrotemporal analysis, which is carried out in the auditory cortices bilaterally in the supratemporal plane. These spectrotemporal computations appear to differ between the two hemispheres. Phonological level processing and representations involves the middle to posterior portions of the superior temporal gyrus (STG) bilaterally, although there may be weak left-hemisphere bias at this level of processing (Hickok and Poeppel 2007).

On the production side, ("from sound to action"), the dorsal stream maps sensory or phonological representations onto articulatory motor representations. (Fig. 4.5). It comprises a sensory-motor interface at the parieto-temporal junction (parietal-temporal boundary: area Spt), whereas the more anterior location in the frontal lobe, probably involving Broca's area and a more dorsal premotor site, corresponds to parts of the articulatory network (pIFG; PM and anterior, left dominant).

Learning to speak involves from the earliest stage the lower part of the motor strip (rolandic) adjacent to the classical Broca's area. According to Poeppel et al. (2012, p 14126), 'The canonical language region, Broca's area, is now known, based on innovative cytoarchitectural and immunocytochemical data, to be composed of a number of subregions (on the order of 10, ignoring possible laminar specializations), plausibly implicating a much greater number of different functions than previously assumed (Amunts et al. 2010), supporting both language and non-language processing'.

Contribution of the new anatomo-functional model to the understanding of Landau–Kleffner syndrome/epilepsy-aphasia spectrum

Children with LKS have language impairments and modes of evolution that differ from those with childhood aphasias due to acquired focal brain lesions. Even those with late onset of LKS do not present the classic aphasic syndromes reported in adults. LKS represents therefore a unique experiment of nature as the epileptic dysfunction 'dissects' the language networks at different locations and periods, in the absence of any structural lesion.

The Hickok and Poeppel model may help to understand some of the baffling manifestations reported in LKS that the previous models failed to explain.

It can explain that loss of language understanding can also occur with a purely or predominantly right-sided epileptic dysfunction. A disruption of speech – sound processing may affect the understanding of the message it carries, whatever side is more involved (Fig 4.5).

The observation of global aphasia (comprehension and expression affected simultaneously) that can occur suddenly in some patients with LKS with only temporal posterior involvement can also be better understood with the new model: The epileptic dysfunction

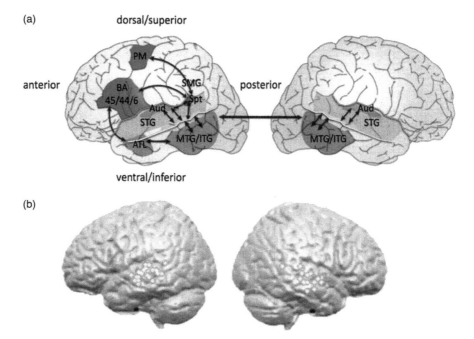

Fig. 4.5. Functional anatomy of language processing dual stream model (from Hickock and Poeppel 2007; Hickock 2009) and phonological aspects of speech perception.

(a). ATL: Anterior temporal lobe; Aud: auditory cortex (early precessing stages); BA 45/44/6: Brodmann areas 45, 44 & 6; MTG/ITG: middle temporal gyrus, inferior temporal gyrus; PM: premotor, dorsal portion; SMG: supramarginal gyrus; Spt: Sylvian parietal temporal region (left only); STG: superior temporal gyrus Sylvian fissure; red line: Sylvian fissure; yellow line: superior temporal sulcus (STS).

(b). Regions associated with phonological aspects of speech perception. Colored dots indicate the distribution of cortical activity from seven studies of speech processing using sublexical stimuli contrasted with various acoustic conditions. Note bilateral distribution centered on the superior temporal sulcus.

can actually involve the Spt area (parietal-temporal junction, dorsal stream) and the middle to posterior portions of the STG (superior temporal sulcus, ventral stream) bilaterally.

Verbal comprehension in patients with LKS can appear very variable, so that it can be mistaken for inattention or unwillingness to respond. An explanation for this can be found in Hickok and Poeppel's statement: 'From a behavioral point of view, it is clear that speech signals contain multiple, partially redundant spectral and temporal cues that can be exploited and that allow speech perception to tolerate a range of signal degradation conditions. This supposes the idea that redundant computational mechanisms, that is parallel processing might exist to exploit these cues'.

The quality of understanding thus depends on the acoustic-perceptual content and the environment in which the oral message is produced, including the source of sounds that cannot be well located. Some words can be understood by recognizing partial linguistic

TABLE 4.1
Remarkable language features observed in some cases of Landau-Kleffner syndrome

Loss of language understanding with a predominant right-side epileptic dysfunction
No clear cut separation between global versus verbal auditory agnosia
Naming difficulties with posterior involvment only
Global aphasia (comprehension and expression) affected simultaneously (acutely)
Poor phonological working memory with intact semantic comprehension
Production deficits may evolve independantly from comprehension deficits

features (vowel pattern, 'tonal gestalt'). Overused or acoustically simple words can be identified by their intonation (prosodic information). Prosodic and contextual clues can thus help some children with VAA to understand or guess what is said, despite poor speech–sound recognition. Older children who have residual representations of words probably resort to 'top-down' processing to interpret spoken messages. Younger children and those with additional cognitive deficits in the social and executive domains may be unable to use these higher level skills.

On the expressive side, speech production impairments (articulation disorder, stuttering and dysprosody) may be due to a localized or more widely propagated epileptic dysfunction in the sensory–motor–articulatory circuits of the dorsal stream. These expressive deficits can occur in isolation or in combination with receptive deficits such as VAA, in addition to those due to lack of auditory feedback (see Chapter 5).

Finally, one must always keep in mind that children with LKS and EAS as a group have a brain organization for language that is different from typically developing children. This can either be due to a constitutional variation/anomaly or to an ongoing epileptic activity in developing language networks, or both (Datta et al. 2013a). This will be further discussed in Chapter 8. This puts some limits on the anatomo-functional correlations that can be made on language in these children, in addition to the fact that the latter is based on adult models.

5
THE DIFFERENT CLINICAL FACETS OF LANDAU–KLEFFNER SYNDROME

This chapter is devoted to an analysis of the two main dimensions of Landau–Kleffner syndrome (LKS): the epilepsy and the language. As an introduction and illustration, we present the case histories of two of our patients followed from childhood to adulthood with completely different clinical presentations and courses that highlight the different facets of LKS and the importance of long-term studies.

Clinical vignettes

INITIAL VERBAL AGNOSIA AND COGNITIVE REGRESSION WITH SEVERE PROLONGED EXPRESSIVE APHASIA

Born in 1966, Michel became mute at the age of 5, unable to understand speech and severely cognitively impaired. Six months later, he presented a few nocturnal seizures. His electroencephalogram (EEG, awake) showed frequent bilateral and asynchronous focal epileptic discharges with left-sided predominance. The first considered diagnosis was a progressive illness, possibly a chronic encephalitis. A few weeks later, he was mainly profoundly aphasic but still could understand many situations around him when verbal language was not required. Language comprehension improved rapidly, but he had a long-standing isolated expressive language impairment with mild oromotor apraxia. Seizures did not recur. He never received steroids. Michel is now 48 years old, and we are still in contact with him. He works as a driver in a car company and lives a fully independent life (details can be found in the original publication (Deonna 1977) and in our book (Deonna and Roulet-Perez 2005) under the initials MR.

Figure 5.1 summarizes the course of the disorder: After a brief phase of receptive language deficit and more global cognitive impairment, his language disorder turned out to be a long-standing isolated expressive speech impairment with mild permanent residual oromotor apraxia. Both were definitely acquired, because he had no developmental speech or oromotor difficulties before the onset of the disease.

Michel's story is not that of the typical isolated VAA (Rapin et al. 1977), which is the emblematic language disorder of LKS, and was for a long time considered a defining feature. We now know that the 'aphasia' in LKS is actually a spectrum with variable involvement of speech and language functions, sometimes associated with other cognitive and behavioural impairments.

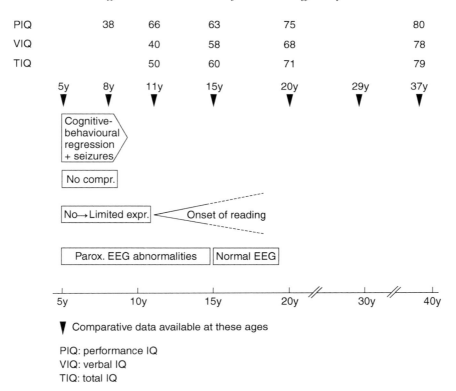

Fig. 5.1. Michel: Long-term cognitive and language evolution from 5 to 40 years. Compr., comprehension; expr., expression; Parox., paroxysmal. From Deonna and Roulet-Perez, Cognitive and Behavioural Disorders of Epileptic Origin in Children. Clinics in Developmental Medicine No. 168. London: Mac Keith Press 2005, p 202.

SEVERE GLOBAL AUDITORY AGNOSIA WITH A SHORT COURSE – 'HE TOLD US THE WHOLE STORY'

Gerard, a boy born in 1988, was in speech therapy for an isolated articulation disorder. A fully normal language examination (audio-taped) was obtained just before he presented with a gradual almost complete loss of language comprehension at the age of 5 years 3 months. This occurred within 3 months and included non-verbal sounds. Verbal expression deteriorated: Speech was fast and halting with poorly articulated and distorted words (inversions, simplifications and omissions of syllables) and naming difficulties. The mother also mentioned that he had lost his strong regional accent. The diagnosis of LKS was made at the age of 6. His EEG showed bilateral independent foci of focal sharp waves in the central region (only 12 electrodes) activated by sleep, but without CSWS. Language was assessed during a 3-day hospital stay and later regularly, first during a 6-week unsuccessful therapy with clobazam and later during rapid improvement with oral prednisone (first improvement after only one week of therapy). Prednisone was given for half a year because of persistent, even if much decreased, epileptiform discharges. Comparative language evaluations and a detailed interview, as soon as he could express himself more easily allowed to document

35

short term fluctuation of his word comprehension (from one day to another), with the feeling of becoming intermittently deaf and the presence of auditory hallucinations (scary noises) (see Fig 5.2). He had no behavioural problems. He fully recovered within a few months except the mild articulatory disorder (substitution of /k/ by /t/) he had before disease onset and a complete right ear extinction on dichotic listening. Importantly, he reported right hemifacial nocturnal seizures that had gone unnoticed and that he drew spontaneously (see Fig 5.2). These had started for some months before the onset of the aphasia and recurred in clusters for the next 4 years without relapse of the language deficit. He has always been an excellent student with good written language and at the age of 23, completed an engineering course successfully.

G's open personality, his parent's willingness to collaborate and his rapid recovery were a gift that allowed us to document most facets of LKS. The occurrence of rolandic seizures long before the aphasia and subsequently for 4 years after language recovery suggests that the epileptic dysfunction affected distinct neuronal networks within the perisylvian area across time.

Analysis of the epilepsy and language impairments in LKS

The detailed analysis we now present is based on the numerous case reports found in the literature. These obviously represent a selection and reporting bias. The fact that these cases were published means that the speech-language impairment was of sufficient severity and duration to be studied. There are good reasons to believe that minor degrees of the same symptoms can occur more frequently than believed and pass unnoticed or explained otherwise.

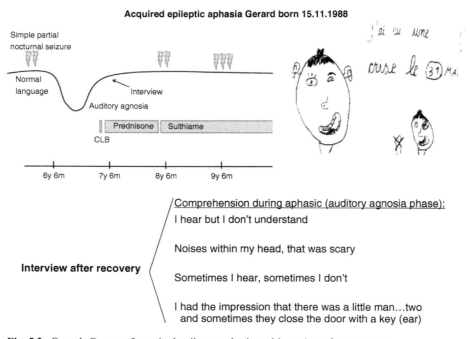

Fig. 5.2. Gerard: Course of acquired epilepsy aphasia and interview after recovery.

We will distinguish (1) the epilepsy, that is the seizures themselves (electroencephalo-gram [EEG] is discussed in Chapter 9); (2) the dynamics of language deficits that reflects their functional epileptic nature and (3) the nature of the speech – language deficits in its variability and combinations.

Analysis of the epileptic and motor manifestations of LKS

EPILEPTIC SEIZURES

A disproportionate importance has naturally been devoted to the description of seizures, their response to therapy and evolution, because this is what neurologists and epileptologists mainly deal with. Suppression of seizures was initially considered of utmost importance, much more than is the case now. This was often achieved easily, mainly because seizures are rare in this syndrome. These are mostly diurnal or nocturnal focal sensorimotor or apparently generalized motor seizures. Children with frequent or multiple seizure types such as myclonic, atonic seizures, atypical absences or focal seizures with altered awareness are the exception in LKS.

LKS WITH ACQUIRED GLOBAL OR UNILATERAL MOTOR DEFICITS

Some authors (Neville et al. 1998) insist on motor impairments such as falls, ataxia and clumsiness, that seem to start, fluctuate and remit along with the language deficit. This is in keeping with some parent's reports of acquired clumsiness in the acute phase. Changes in handedness have also been reported. These motor disturbances have not been systemati-cally studied and could have several causes : direct seizure-related motor deficits such as 'negative myoclonus' or epileptic 'pseudoataxia' due to constant subclinical myclonic jerks causing disequilibrium (as in children with ABPE; see discussion on classification), body scheme or proprioceptive sensory deficits, apraxia, hemineglect (Maquet et al. 1995; Paquier et al. 2009), or inattention and impulsiveness leading to falls.

Considering the now large number of reported children with LKS, the rarity of motor and sensory deficits, except oromotor deficits, supports the notion that the epilepstogenic and propagation zones are generally limited to the perisylvian regions. Limb or more global motor impairments are mainly seen in other epilepsy-aphasia syndromes (EAS) such as acquired epileptic opercular syndrome (AEOS) and ABPE.

FOCAL AUDITORY SEIZURES

It is expected that epileptic activity in the auditory cortex could generate in addition to loss of function 'positive' manifestations in the form of auditory distortions or elementary audi-tory hallucinations, by analogy with other focal epilepsies arising in the temporal neocor-tex, such as the syndrome of autosomal dominant epilepsy with auditory features (Winaver et al. 2000). There are of course very limited data on that possibility in children with LKS, because the children cannot express themselves. When they recover, most often many months or years later, they may not remember or are not asked about it. The child with a brief period of auditory agnosia (GA described above) told us that he heard 'noises within my head, that was scary'. At the same period he also mentioned that 'from time to time I could not hear'. Morrell et al. (1995), while performing prolonged electrophysiological studies in children with LKS who were candidates for epilepsy surgery (see Chapters 10 and 12) mentioned that:

> video-monitoring had proved to be extremely valuable because many patients have seizures that are often subtle and often missed by the family. Sometimes only subjective behavioral manifestations are described as 'roaring in my ears sounds like a lion', and are accompanied by covering both ears with the hands. Such phenomena have been found to be correlated with electrographic seizure discharges. Descriptions such as those were obtained when the seizures began and before the onset of aphasia or, rarely, after recovery as they are remembered, but the gesture of suddenly covering the ears with a terrified expression is something that can be seen even in those children who are already mute.

These observations signify that focal auditory seizures manifesting as periods of hearing loss, auditory distortion or elementary auditory hallucinations can occur in LKS and go unnoticed or are interpreted as behavioural disorders. These paroxysmal ictal events have to be distinguished from the prolonged aphasic manifestations that electrographically do not correspond with seizure activity *per se* (see Chapter 10).

One should stress here that the clinical recognition of epileptic seizures depends on the function of the cortex from which they start and propagate. Rolandic seizures or other motor seizures or those with impairment of awareness or autonomic symptoms are easily identified as there is a clear, acute disruption of normal neural function. When a seizure involves a network sub-serving a specific cognitive skill (e.g. listening, speaking or reading), it will remain unrecognized, unless the child is actively involved in a task requiring its use.

TIME CORRELATION BETWEEN SEIZURES AND LANGUAGE DEFICIT

Only a minority of children present with simultaneous onset of seizures and language disturbances. Most had seizures, sometimes long before the onset of the language deficit. Others start having seizures months or years after the aphasia sets in. Some children never had any seizures, a proportion that increased as LKS became more and more recognized, now estimated at about 30% of cases. Fluctuations, remissions and exacerbations of the aphasia often seem independent from the presence of seizures. Seizures can relapse months or years after the aphasia has resolved or has much improved but this is not necessarily associated with a new language regression. These data have long been wrongly taken as an argument that the aphasia is not directly related to the epilepsy, but a manifestation of an unknown underlying brain disease.

Dynamics of installation and evolution of language (fluctuations) in children with LKS

One of the main arguments that LKS is based on an epileptic process – regardless of its underlying mechanisms – is the extraordinarily variable dynamics in the installation, course, progression and presence of long-term chronic deficits. Antiepileptic therapy, for the better or the worse, can of course account for these variable evolutions, although there are clearly children with spontaneous acute, subacute, slow, very slow onset and recovery (see Chapter 10).

The difficulty of providing precise pieces of information on the dynamics of language loss and its correlations with epilepsy variables has been and remains a major issue. Understandably, severe cases, which are more likely to be reported, are studied when the situation is stable or improving, that is, when the child is willing or capable of cooperating and rarely at the peak of the disease when immediate medical diagnostic and therapeutic concerns are in the forefront. In mild cases, there may be delay in diagnosis, because intermittent inaccurate comprehension of language or unclear, repetitive, slurred or stuttering speech, is difficult to interpret in young children. A father who filmed his daughter as soon as the epilepsy started wrote the following in a personal letter to TD:

> *Since we had not been aware of speech deterioration until it was too notorious, we were astonished to look back to recordings and not having noticed it before! It's been very useful to trace a line between what seemed to be a normal language development and then abnormal language (stuttering, non-word language and silentness) to try to figure out when the illness started.*

Furthermore, the other associated intermittent deficits, such as major inattention, withdrawal or cognitive regression that can occur as the epilepsy worsens can render language evaluation very difficult.

The onset of the language deficit may be abrupt ('overnight') or insidious and slowly progressive. It may also be initially abrupt but with later slower aggravation, or the reverse, and this sometimes in a same child. Recovery can also be rapid or gradual. Sometimes, there is no recovery at all. These symptom dynamics may be seen at different epochs, months or years apart with a great variability in severity of language impairment at any point independently of therapy Remissions and exacerbations can occur for several years, at unpredictable intervals from the time of the original initial episode. Exacerbations tend to get less and less severe and frequent until final remission occurs. This represents essentially the natural history of the disorder. In the first 20 to 30 years after the recognition of LKS, EEGs, especially during sleep, were not regularly performed in children if there was no seizure relapse. In addition, most children received classic antiepileptic drugs such as carbamazepine, phenobarbital or phenytoine, used in focal epilepsies, which could worsen the epilepsy and specifically increase the interictal epileptiform discharges (IEDs).

Interestingly, spontaneous marked fluctuations have always been noted and were well described in some of the old reports of children who received no AEDs (Pötzl 1926; Jakab 1950). It is surprising that these striking variations in the severity of aphasia were not more emphasized upon, since besides epilepsy, few neurological disorders except migraine or remitting-relapsing inflammatory diseases may present such dynamics. Rapin et al.'s (1977) article entitled 'Acquired verbal auditory agnosia in children' case 1 well illustrates these major fluctuations in the severity of the language disorder with also variable EEG findings. Both insidious and rapid regressions and recovery and also transient worsening of speech after a seizure (Todd's like) were observed. Figure 5.3 has been drawn from the case report and, according to the author, corresponds well with her observations (I Rapin, personal communication, 2012).

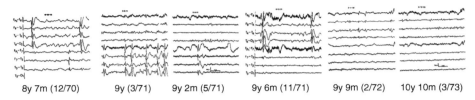

| 8y 7m (12/70) | 9y (3/71) | 9y 2m (5/71) | 9y 6m (11/71) | 9y 9m (2/72) | 10y 10m (3/73) |

① 8y 7m : Difficulty with speech comprehension and complains he could not hear; spoke less and less

② 9y 7m : Suddenly improved over two weeks. Amount of spontaneous speech increased dramatically and comprehension returned to normal

③ 10y 1m : Relapse for a few weeks. "Marked difficulty understanding speech and repeating words".

④ 11y : Normal neuropsychological and language evaluation. Persistent articulatory disorder.

1a: Two months later his mother reported a generalized seizure followed by transient worsening of speech

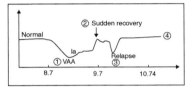

Fig. 5.3. Major fluctuations in a seminal case of Landau–Kleffner syndrome (VAA, verbal auditory agnosia). Adapted from Rapin et al. 1977.

Two other case reports in the literature illustrate in a spectacular way the recurrent fluctuating course of the aphasia.

RECURRENT GLOBAL AGNOSIA IN LKS

Luat et al. (2006) reported a 4-year-old child with five episodes of 'typical isolated auditory agnosia' over an 18-month period, each one of 3 weeks duration with intermittent difficulties in comprehension in the first week, worsening during the second week and return to normal during the third week (between episodes; PIQ:112, VIQ: 88). This was certainly the natural evolution of the disorder as it occurred under unchanged monotherapy with oxcarbazepine (Fig 5.4).

The fluctuating language impairment can result from successful antiepileptic therapy with spectacular remissions. Worsening may also be drug induced, a situation that is not easy to recognize, because it is rarely immediate. When the language deficit is severe and has been of long duration, some improvement in language comprehension may be very difficult to document and may come after a long delay, after the EEG has already normalized, for reasons that are complex and ill understood (see Chapters 9 and 10).

SEVERE PROLONGED ACQUIRED APHASIA WITHOUT FLUCTUATIONS AND RECOVERY

There are patients with profound, prolonged or permanent aphasia in whom no recovery takes place and no fluctuation are seen, even when the epileptiform discharges disappeared or decreased significantly. These patients challenged the notion that the aphasia

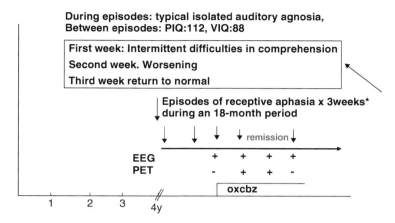

Fig. 5.4. Episodic receptive aphasia in a child with Landau–Kleffner syndrome. (Adapted from Luat et al., 2006.)

is a functional disorder with the same underlying pathophysiology as the less severe and fluctuating cases (Kaga 1999). These severe cases were mainly children with LKS of early onset, with pre-existing language impairment and/or delayed diagnosis. They did not receive therapy, or if they did, it was given late (months or years) after the first symptoms. In some of these, the EEG discharges persisted despite therapy, including steroids and epilepsy surgery. This pattern of evolution will be further discussed in Chapter 7.

UNEXPECTED TRANSIENT IMPROVEMENT IN THE COURSE OF LONG-STANDING SEVERE DEFICITS
These seemingly anecdotal and poorly documented observations of unexpected transient improvement in long-standing severe deficits have the last place in this list of patterns of language evolution in LKS. It is difficult to conclude if these 'unbelievable' observations were real or the product of wishful thinking. Such cases are sometimes informally discussed in international meetings but never published. Two anecdotal experiences of one the author (TD) are worth mentioning here: In an old correspondence with a teacher from the Institution for the Deaf where one of our patients with profound longstanding auditory agnosia and limited speech resided, I found the following note: 'One morning, after a seizure the day before, he had a day of brief and apparently spectacular improvement of his language'. I asked the staff to let me know immediately if it would happen again, but it never did. The other is in a brief note from a case report published by Glos et al. (2001) on a child with LKS and a longstanding auditory agnosia and global regression: 'Twice, immediately after awakening, the girl was able to communicate orally for 2 minutes' (see case report 2, Lanzi et al. 1994, p47).

Figure 5.5 summarizes the main possible courses and different dynamics of the language disorder drawn from case histories of the now hundreds of children described in the

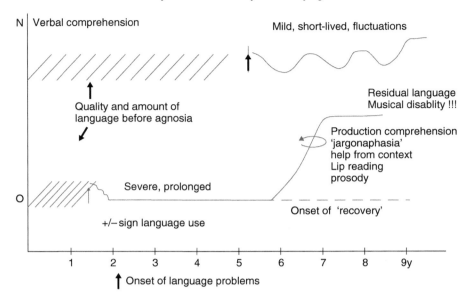

Fig. 5.5. Contrasted trajectories of different LKS cases. It illustrates cases of late onset, mild course and rapid improvement (upper curve) while others have an early onset , and severe protracted course (lower curve). N, normal language verbal comprehension. 0, absent verbal comprehension.

literature on LKS (mainly VAA). They are certainly biased in favour of the most severe cases and are independent from the seizure history, which is often more detailed than the language symptoms. It appears now that the dichotomy between early onset, gradual prolonged course and the later onset, more acute, fluctuating, briefer and less severe course, as depicted in the figure is somewhat artificial. There are many more variations in the timing, nature and evolution of symptoms, including purely expressive deficits between different children and in the a same child. It is possible that severe cases will be less and less frequent with earlier recognition and therapy.

Types of language deficits

Table 5.1 illustrates how the mode of onset and nature of the language deficits can influence the way they are interpreted (first complaints and main reasons), the observed modes of evolution, the suspected level of neuropsychological impairment and how the deficits are often named or categorized. It can be seen (comment in the table) how one has started from the restricted view of 'LKS = auditory agnosia' to the other later recognized predominant speech and language deficits reflecting the main location of the epileptic activity within the perisylvian region.

Note that this table does not incorporate the deficits that would start very early on in life and come to attention as a 'developmental' speech or language delay.

TABLE 5.1

Variety of initial manifestations, evolving patterns and range and nature of functional deficits reported in Landau–Kleffner syndrome

First and chief complaint	Main explanation	Evolution	Corresponding neuropsychological – neurological deficit	Level of impairment	Comments
Speech perception: 'deaf', 'inattentive', 'not responding', 'oppositional'	Difficulties with verbal comprehension	Intermittent or recurrent sound /speech perception difficulties; Progressive total absence of response to sound; Gradual or simultaneous deterioration of production ('speech loss')	Auditory agnosia; Verbal auditory agnosia (VAA) or global auditory agnosia; Other comprehension deficits (lexical, semantic)	Phonologic discrimination (or other specific acoustic features of words)	Considered most common 'typical LKS'; Initial global auditory agnosia can evolve into verbal auditory agnosia; When good recovery, often residual subtle speech–sound discrimination difficulties
Speech arrest: 'stops speaking and responding' (rapid)	Complete loss of comprehension and mutism	No recovery; Progressive slow recovery (months/years) Recovery, partial, fluctuations	Total agnosia of VAA, combined word finding problems (anomia) or other expressive deficits	Phonologic decoding Articulatory networks (auditory motor programming)	Selective mutism or other psychological disorder can be suspected
Deterioration of speech: 'speaks less' 'slow speech' 'garbled speech' 'jargon', 'unintelligible'	Impairment at different levels of speech production	Progression to total speech loss; Fluctuations with intermittent recovery; Impairment of comprehension	Articulation disorder*; Stuttering; Dysfluency; Dysprosody; Naming problems (anomia)* most prominent, often combinations	Several levels of speech productionprograms (from word conceptualization to articulatory features of words)	Expressive and mixed forms of LKS; Expressve difficulties often under-recognized; Can antedate onset of comprehension deficits, hence unexplained by loss of auditory feedback of speech
Oromotor problems: 'difficulty eating' 'drooling' 'unclear speech'	Impairment of voluntary movements of bulbar musculature	Severe oromotor paralysis('tube-fed'); Fluctuations, recovery Residual speech articulation deficits	Oromotor apraxia Suprabulbar paralysis	Motor execution of buccolingofacial (non-linguistic) movements	Now referred to as acquired epileptic opercular syndrome; Full or significant recovery even in severe cases, residual apraxia of speech/dysarthria in cases with familial forms

From auditory agnosia to verbal auditory agnosia

An isolated global auditory or verbal auditory agnosia may occur initially while spontaneous expressive speech is still present, but impairment may be noticed when the child has to repeat a word or sentence that he has understood only partially or with distortions. Progressively, speech becomes unintelligible leading to mutism with a few remaining simple and over-learned productions. This is believed to be the most typical scenario, with the suspicion of deafness being the first parental complaint. A complete simultaneous loss of comprehension and expression, either abrupt or gradual, is much more rarely reported and suggests global aphasia due to a more extensive dysfunction of the language networks. Nevertheless, according to Hickock and Poeppel's model, a localized disruption in the Spt region can also explain global aphasia (see Chapter 4).

The long-prevailing opinion has been that impaired verbal comprehension in LKS is secondary to a phonologic discrimination and processing impairment (Metz-Lutz 2009). If the impairment is severe, comprehension will be impossible. If it is partial, it will mainly affect less frequent words that cannot be 'guessed' like more common ones. The phonologic short-term memory span and verbal working memory are also impaired, and this will affect sentence comprehension, new word acquisition and written language learning. It is nevertheless remarkable that some children with a poor verbal-auditory memory after they have recovered from LKS can understand rather complex messages, because sufficient information has reached the lexical-semantic store, enough to get the meaning of a request to carry out an action or to retell a story in one's own words (Majerus et al. 2004).

At the peak of the disorder, children may lose the ability to recognize the meaning of environmental sounds and even locate their source (auditory agnosia). At this level of severity, the response to sounds is typically inconsistent, probably because the child learns to ignore meaningless auditory information. However, there are sometimes definite reactions to sounds, mainly in natural settings. As a parent quoted on an American website on LKS put it, 'I can't tell you how many times I have had to convince teachers that my child is not deaf'.

When they improve, the children start again to recognize common environmental sounds, whereas they do not recognize most words, because the complexity of their acoustic features. However, short words composed of a short vowel or a stop (or plosive) consonant (such as p, k and t) can be in a given context recognized as a word belonging to the child's previous repertoire (see Chapter 4). Figure 5.6 shows the schematic recovery from global agnosia to full comprehension, an evolution that has been repeatedly described, but rarely measured (Korkman et al. 1998).

Non-verbal sounds of high complexity can sometimes be recognized when no decoding of phonemes or words is possible. This has been taken as evidence of a higher level phonologic discrimination deficit in LKS (Korkman et al. 1998). See also Chapter 4.

Higher level language deficits affecting lexicon or syntax can be found when recovery of basic word comprehension at the level of the word is sufficient to be assessed. The reasons for a longstanding incomplete comprehension of discourse are probably multifold. Different levels of auditory/verbal processing can be affected with recovery occurring at various rates over time. There may be short-term fluctuating levels of the epileptic

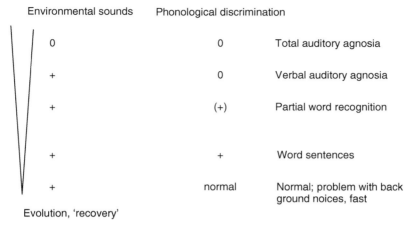

Fig. 5.6. Recovery from global auditory agnosia. Absence of any auditory recognition (0) to gradual recognition (+) of environmental sounds and later phonologic discrimination as seen in severe cases.

dysfunction, especially in cases of recent onset or in phases of improvement or exacerbations with the child regressing to global auditory agnosia again (Kaga 1999). These explain why it can be so difficult to precisely assess the child's abilities. The extent of the deficit in language comprehension can be either over- or underestimated; the latter occurs more often because contextual prosodic or visual clues (lip reading) can sometimes be sufficient for significant comprehension. Finally, an intercurrent conductive hearing loss associated with throat or middle ear infection (glue ears) may alter the quality of auditory information reaching a recovering auditory network and can be mistaken for a relapse of LKS.

DISSOCIATION BETWEEN COMPREHENSION AND EXPRESSION
Speech problems encountered in children with LKS are not only the consequence of degraded auditory input similar to what is observed in acquired deafness (the earlier the worse the outcome), as initially thought.

In acquired deafness, expression depends on normal auditory feedback, the more so that language has been recently learned. This was Bishop's conclusion about LKS in her study on the impact of age at onset of VAA on outcome and has been accepted for a long time since (Bishop 1985). However, Bishop also mentioned the following:

It would seem that in at least some cases of LKS, the language problems cannot be totally explained as secondary symptoms arising from a primary auditory processing disorder. If it is the case that the language areas of the brain are operating normally but are simply receiving defective auditory input, one might expect pronunciation to deteriorate, but the child should not forget words he previously knew. In fact word finding problems are a frequent feature of the language disorder in children with onset above age 7 years.

Expressive deficits are actually variable in LKS, both at onset, during the course of the disorder and after recovery, and this has not been extensively studied. Total speech loss may be the first symptom while verbal comprehension is still present to a fair degree or even normal, and when it improves, major word finding difficulties can appear. Articulation is most often distorted very early on and disturbances of speech fluency – stuttering, prolonged pauses filled with unusual vocalization and sometimes a 'foreign accent syndrome' (FAS; see below) can be observed. These may be speech deficits on their own, possibly unrelated to the degree of comprehension. They can also fluctuate and change in the course of the disorder.

The possible dissociation between production and comprehension was a surprise when we looked at some old but precise longitudinal case descriptions. It is well in keeping with recent data on language organization (see the Hickok and Poeppel model in Chapter 4) and specifically speech perception. This is also congruent with the focal, but often changing sites and spread of the epileptic dysfunction in the course of the disorder.

There are two exceptional case reports in the literature demonstrating this dissociation between expression and comprehension. Interestingly, this was not the main point of either paper. However, it was evident when looking into the details. We have adapted the data presented in the Figure 5.7 from the original text with the authors' permission (Lanzi et al. 1994).

Case 1 Mariën et al. (1993) published a longitudinal study of a boy who had onset of speech production and comprehension difficulties at the age of 4 years and 2 months and slowly regressed to the point of complete mutism and auditory agnosia at the age of 5 years and 9 months. The authors who first met him at 5 years and 8 months made a diagnosis of LKS and started intensive speech and language therapy as well as AED treatment. Despite all these, the deficit evolved to a global aphasia within 1 month. After 3 months, language started to improve. At 5 years and 11 months, the child had recovered sufficient language, so that a quantitative analysis of several dimensions of production and comprehension could be performed. A longitudinal evaluation was then carried out monthly or bimonthly from 5 years and 11 months to 6 years and 7 months. Close follow-up showed marked fluctuations of language skills with improvement and again regression. At one point, however, spontaneous speech started to deteriorate, with an increase of 'motor aphasic symptomatology', while auditory and verbal comprehension for both words and sentences was gradually improving. Only 2 months later did auditory verbal comprehension deteriorate again.

Case 2 Lanzi et al. (1994), assessed speech production and comprehension longitudinally and quantitatively at several successive periods when their patient either relapsed or improved in correlation with the EEG epileptiform discharges and therapy (the latter was the point of the paper).

There were eight comparative examinations from age 4 years and 6 months until 6 years and 10 months. Comprehension was tested with a sentence-matching task (compared with typically developing children) and production with mean length of utterance (MLU) and analysis of phonologic alterations. At onset, the child had

> absence of structured language, onomatopeic sounds and absence of verbal comprehension. At 6.2 years, there was a relapse with a severe drop in verbal comprehension

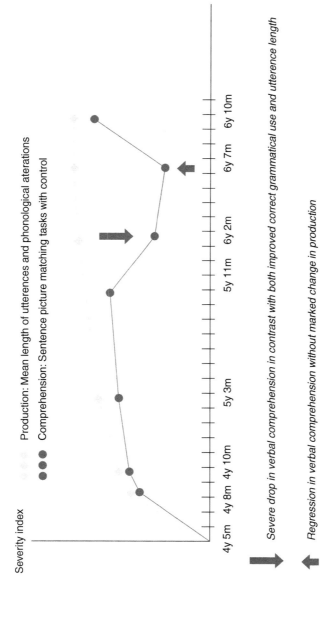

Fig. 5.7. Dissociation between production and comprehension. (Created from data in Lanzi et al., 1994)

in contrast with both improved grammatical use and utterance length as compared to results at 4.10 and 5.3 years. At 6.7 years, there was a further 'relapse in verbal comprehension without marked change in production'. A clear dissociation of the level of production (which was maintained) from the level of verbal comprehension (which recorded a dramatic drop) was mentioned.

As this finding was not the main message of the paper, it was not mentioned in the abstract!

Both cases show that expressive and receptive deficit can coexist or have a dissociated course that can pass completely unnoticed if fluctuations are not major and are not looked at closely. The dissociated course indicates that the expressive deficits are not necessarily the consequence of the receptive deficit. It illustrates the epileptic nature of the language dysfunction and how the epileptic process can 'dissect' the different components and levels of the complex language networks modelled by Hickok and Poeppel (see Chapter 4).

Other types of aphasic symptoms in LKS

The use of a narrow definition of LKS taking VAA as a major criterion that most clinicians have adopted can explain that other types of acquired language deficits have escaped recognition or description. Chevrie-Muller et al. (1991) in a team of linguists and paediatric neurologists reported a 'peculiar case of LKS' with a long follow-up from 4 years and 6 months to 11 years with 'verbal-auditory unawareness and neglect with partial comprehension' and a major difficulty in naming with pauses filled with song-like vocalization. Their careful review of LKS-reported cases showed that several children had linguistic features other than VAA with its consequences on speech production.

ACQUIRED LEXICAL-SEMANTIC APHASIA IN THE FRAME OF AN EAS SYNDROME

This is, to our knowledge, a so far unreported evolution of a child with an atypical form of rolandic epilepsy with severe seizures and CSWS (corresponding to ABPE) whose precisely documented linguistic evolution allowed documentation of another type of comprehension deficit within the EAS spectrum (Allen 2016).

This boy was followed from age 1 year and 11 months when he had his first rolandic seizure, up to the age of 13 years. His brain MRI was normal. He subsequently developed oromotor difficulties, refractory multiple seizure types and a global cognitive and language regression coincident with CSWS on the EEG. The epilepsy was finally controlled with steroids. Longitudinal follow-up showed a specific lexical–semantic deficit language impairment (both in comprehension and in production) along with a moderate global cognitive deficit and communication difficulties within the autistic spectrum disorder (ASD).

SPEECH PRODUCTION DEFICITS AND MUTISM IN LKS

As discussed above, there has been an enormous publication bias to only report cases of LKS with VAA because this was understood as a diagnostic criterion. The onset of the language disorder was often not studied or data about this period were not available. However, the review of all cases in the literature in which some details were given (usually anecdotal and 'naïve' descriptions) revealed that 'mutism' and 'total loss of speech' could occur when comprehension was still preserved. When the child had no seizures and no oromotor difficulties (drooling and swallowing problems), it is not surprising that mutism was initially considered of psychological origin. This is what happened in the following case by Koupernik et al. (1969).

This 5-year-old girl lost speech 4–5 months after a sexual assault. (Koupernik et al. 1969). The speech problems started as 'paroxysmal anarthric episodes', difficulty with articulation, followed by a total loss of speech. She used gestures and always wanted to communicate. She also had paroxysmal sleep episodes considered as night terrors. It is unclear if she understood speech or auditory stimuli at this time. It was never discussed that she might have become deaf. Two years later it was mentioned that 'repetition and naming were impossible'. She had several EEGs interpreted as normal initially, but 2 years later, she developed status epilepticus and a right focal motor seizure was recorded on the EEG. A sleep tracing a month later showed 'spike activity in the left temporal area' (J. Roger, Marseille). In retrospect, one can interpret this case as LKS, with an initial fluctuating isolated problem in speech production (anarthria and articulation problems) followed some time later by auditory agnosia. Interestingly, she had a speech spectrogram by a renowned physician and speech pathologist (Dr. Claude Chevrie-Muller) showing that 'intonation and rhythm of the vocal productions were very particular "with syllabic repetition and prolonged holding of the vowel"'…'These sounds do not evoke the babbling of the young child… They have a bizarre pattern' (Koupernik et al. 1969). This patient may have been the first electrophysiologically recorded sample of a severely distorted and rather unique acquired speech pathology in LKS initially considered of psychological origin. The authors interpreted their case as Hellers' dementia (see Chapter 2), noting also that 'the role of the psychic trauma could not be denied'. They finally acknowledged its resemblance to those described by Worster-Drought (1971): 'an unusual form of acquired aphasia in children'.

In less severe cases, mention is often made of 'slow speech', 'stuttering', 'dysfluency', various types of articulatory problems (with sometimes 'groping efforts with the mouth before a word is produced', at the phonemic, syllabic or whole word level), 'naming problems', word finding difficulty in spontaneous discourse, changes in the child's usual prosody and 'loss of native accent' or 'sounding like a foreign accent'. These difficulties sometimes worsened to what is globally described as 'dilapidated speech', 'garbled speech' or 'totally unintelligible speech'. For instance, in the paper by Dulac et al. (1983), 4 out of 10 children had initially expressive deficits: 'dysarthria' and ' paraphasia' (1 child), 'expressive problems' (2 children), 'impoverishment of expression' (1 child). More than one of these diverse production problems could be present in the same child or develop in the course of the disorder, articulation difficulties being the most frequently reported.

These various clinical descriptions suggest different and possibly very specific dysfunctions along the dorsal stream ('from sound to action'; see Hickok and Poeppel (2007) in Chapter 4).

ISOLATED PRODUCTION DEFICIT EVOLVING TO PROLONGED MUTISM

An exceptionally well-documented situation in which an isolated production deficit progressing to complete mutism contrasting with normal comprehension has been studied by

Gunilla Rejnö-Habte Selassie and Paul Uvebrandt (unpublished) and is reported in some detail in Chapter 15.

<small>THE PLACE OF PSYCHOLOGICAL SPEECH INHIBITION IN CASES OF MUTISM IN THE CONTEXT</small>
OF LKS

We know how speech production can be affected by difficult psychological situations and strong emotions, and how this can be a problem in persons, especially in children who do not master speech and language well for various reasons such as having to learn a foreign language and in children with developmental language disorder (DLD).

Some children with DLD are particularly sensitive to social or other stressful conversational contexts. They experience from their speech distortions, syntactic weaknesses and slowness of exchanges that they know are much aggravated in demanding conversations. Typically, for those with word retrieval problems, having to answer specific questions or tell a precise story is the most difficult and is therefore avoided.

In children with acquired speech and language impairments like in LKS, this situation is even worse when they have experienced that their ability to speak is unpredictable (epileptic fluctuations). They may feel powerless, unwilling or incapable to try to speak, knowing that their need/desire to communicate depends on a tool they cannot master properly. In many circumstances, the child may feel 'better to shut up'. The result is that a component of speech inhibition or selective mutism – that is, present in some social circumstances – may add to the underlying disorder, rendering it more difficult to assess and follow-up.

<small>PROSODY IN</small> LKS

It is known from adult neurology studies that prosody can be specifically lost in comprehension or in expression as a result of diverse brain injuries, and there are rare reports of isolated and temporary loss of the prosodic aspects of speech in focal epilepsy (Deonna et al. 1987). Understanding of verbal messages by the child from very early on in life depends on prosody before the decoding of the exact meaning of a word (semantics) is understood. Prosody or 'melody of speech' refers to acoustic features of speech (such as intonation, pitch, tempo, volume and timbre). These features are called 'suprasegmental' as opposed to 'segmental', referring to phonemes. Prosody conveys essential and quite different pieces of information from words, that is ,the intention and states of mind of the speaker, mostly with a communicative intent. An important distinction has been made in recent years between linguistic prosody and affective prosody. Linguistic prosody refers to how a specific linguistic information (question form, declaration and demand) is conveyed by changes in tone, loudness, rhythm etc.). Affective prosody refers to the verbal expression of emotional states produced by playing on different vocal and other acoustic aspects of speech. In routine exchanges, much of what is going on can be understood, with the aid of context, by this dimension of speech and may be relied upon when the knowledge of precise meaning of words is missing (like with a foreign language), lost or distorted (like in VAA).

In LKS, it has been largely assumed that the loss of the perception of acoustic characteristics of phonemes and higher level of phonological processing was enough to account for all communication difficulties. An alteration or on the contrary a preservation of prosody was not seriously considered. Parents sometimes mention that their child lost her/his local accent and had developed a foreign accent or a robotic speech. This could be transient and apparently could happen before or independently from the loss of comprehension or expression. It suggests that prosody was affected, but this topic has been largely untouched. Doherty et al. (1999) showed that prosody was preserved in two patients with LKS. These authors suggested that one should consider taking advantage of that for language rehabilitation. However, prosody was not assessed formally and the distinction between linguistic and affective prosody was not made. We met a 25-year-old woman with a late diagnosed global auditory agnosia acquired in early childhood who had no recovery (case 2, Van Bogaert et al. 2013). She does watch movies on television with earphones to the surprise of the family and obviously gets some information from the protagonist's emotional prosody.

Kim Dufor et al. (2012) have studied prosody in three patients with LKS. This followed a major work of standardization and creation of tests in typically developing French-speaking children at increasing ages and in typical adults. The development of the different characteristics of prosody (affective and linguistic) was well documented. Two children and one adolescent with LKS were compared with 7–8-year-old healthy children and healthy adults. Affective prosody was better used in these children than in the control group with the reservation that the patients had relatively late age at onset, short duration of epilepsy/medication and preserved comprehension. No generalization could be made from this small study in which case histories (age at onset, severity, therapy, etc.) and results on prosody tests differed markedly. Interestingly, however, an 8-year-old girl was capable of differentiating between anger and neutral stimuli even in the absence of semantic information, better than the typically developing children who needed it for perception and identification of emotions. She seemed to take advantage of an intact affective prosody.

The standardized and broad test battery created by Kim-Dufor et al. (2012) on all important aspects of prosody in children could certainly be used in new or still evolving cases of LKS (recovering or deteriorating). It could show if and how this dimension of verbal communication is dissociated from others and evolves along with the other linguistic parameters. If affected in an individual child, it may serve as a clinical marker of evolution, probably easier to assess and interpret than verbal tests with test-retest effects.

LOSS OF REGIONAL ACCENT AND FOREIGN ACCENT SYNDROME

Foreign accent syndrome (FAS), described in adults, is defined as a pronunciation by a patient that is perceived by listeners of the same language community as distinctly foreign. It can occur after focal brain lesions mainly of vascular origin. We are not aware that it has been described in children after an acquired brain insult, although it has been rarely reported in DLD (Chevrie-Muller et al. 2007, Marien et al. 2009). The loss of the child's previous accent can only be judged by the family and relatives, whereas a new accent can be recognized by members of the same community as not native (i.e. foreign to that region or typical of the distortions that natives of another language make).

The 'translation' of phonologic knowledge to verbal-motor commands can disrupted in several ways, from a motor speech planning disorder, with disrupted oral diadochokinesia, scanned speech or to a lower down execution of the articulatory schemes. What accounts for the FAS has to our knowledge not been formally studied in LKS. However, it seems to be different from the impairment of prosody described sometimes as 'robotic speech' in some case reports. It is also different from speech in patients with severe with residual VAA who have difficulties pronouncing consonants that they do not discriminate well (inaccurate phonologic representations), similar to the speech of the hearing impaired.

Musical abilities in children with LKS

Human beings differ widely in their natural talent, interest and love for music, and this can be dissociated from verbal abilities. It is particularly striking that some individuals with the greatest linguistic abilities, have no interest in music. For example, Sigmund Freud and William James exhibited no emotional response to music (Sacks 2007).

Since the advent of functional imaging, the neuroanatomy of music perception is better understood (Platel et al. 1997). In normal adults, the left hemisphere is specialized in rhythm perception and musical semantic representations (identification and recognition of memories), whereas the right hemisphere handles melody perception (pitch contours and timbre).

In LKS, the focal epileptic dysfunction in the superior temporal region, often spreading locally or to the contralateral region would be expected to disrupt one or several components of music perception.

Musical abilities appear almost universally affected in the active stage of LKS and can be a permanent sequelae. This is probably because of altered perception of one or several of the attributes of sounds and their temporal organization that constitute music, which is more complex than common environmental sounds.

We have not found any publication specifically devoted to this issue, although we have heard repeatedly from parents and read that an affected child became very poor in recognizing melodies or in singing, did not have much interest in music or continued to have problems with music after he had recovered verbal language. We also have often heard that the child had never been good at music or that the family was 'not musical'. Musical ability appears naturally not as a priority in the active phase of LKS and when impaired, it is logically considered as part of the auditory agnosia. Musical skills are also not easily quantified in children. The loss of an acquired skill in this domain is difficult to measure and consequently not published. It is probably not by chance that the only paper addressing musical ability in LKS came from Japan (Kaga 1999), where musical education starts very early and is universal: As stated by the author (M Kaga, personal communication, 2012):

> I suppose impairment of musical ability in LKS is my very discovery and my pure original description. In Japan, many parents want their children to learn musical instruments such as piano and electric organ (we have so many Yamaha music schools in almost every city!) and music is an essential study subject in elementary schools/junior high schools and an elective subject in high schools. Moreover, Karaoke is an original made-in Japan product. Many people often experience Karaoke in their social lives. We often have times to consider about our/their ability and talents in music in our daily lives.

In the four case reports followed from childhood to adulthood, Kaga described temporary impairment of musical abilities in all children during the active phase of LKS; one recovered completely and was 'good at singing songs', and one was permanently affected with 'amusia-auditory agnosia in music', contrasting with a moderate impairment in auditory verbal perception (telephone conversations or meetings with three or more attendants). Case 4 of Kaga actually represents the first reported case of an isolated acquired epileptic musical disability (amusia) as an almost unique sequel of LKS. Acquired amusia in LKS may be another example of how a focal epileptic activity can selectively affect a developing neuronal network in way of specialization.

Considering the importance of music in children's developing social and emotional life, one wonders how the loss of some or all musical skills in a young child who suffers LKS and who possibly has permanent disability in this domain, is experienced. There are understandably no scientific data on this topic. Christine T, a 28-year-old married woman with two children, who had an early and severe form of the disorder, has written a remarkable testimony of her own childhood memories relating to music (confirmed by her parents) and of her present residual difficulties. Her story can be found in Chapter 15 along with questions/reactions to it by one of the authors of this book.

Musical disability has been a so far neglected facet of LKS, a domain that will now be possible to assess also objectively with available tools for evaluating children's musical abilities across age and culture (Peretz et al. 2013; Levêque et al. unpublished). One can make the hypothesis that some children who develop LKS had previous difficulties with music perception, which could be aggravated by the epileptic disorder. This has not to our knowledge been systematically studied, for example, in rolandic epilepsy and in related syndromes in the milder end of the EAS spectrum in which sound and speech perception can also be altered in more subtle ways.

Impairments in reading and writing

There are no systematic analytic group data on written language acquisition, acquired dyslexia and long-term outcome in this domain in children with LKS. Severe impairments during the acute phase and persistence after recovery have to be expected. LKS most often has its onset at age 4–7y when a child normally starts to be exposed to written language at home or at school. Written language has to be systematically taught, and this occurs in a period corresponding often to the peak of the epileptic disease.

Since the most frequent and typical problem in LKS is a difficulty to decode speech sounds, a child's ability to learn to match the visual aspect of a sound (the letter: grapheme) to its oral counterpart (the phoneme), which is the basis of normal acquisition and teaching of reading and writing in alphabetic languages, will logically be affected.

In addition, written language learning may be hampered indirectly. The child has limited auditory comprehension of what is expected from him, a poor attention span, and is discouraged by a difficult and unrewarding task, like for many dyslexic children, but with additional fluctuating and unpredictable capacities. Playful exercises with words (rhymes, songs and rote learning of poems) that facilitate access to written language are not accessible during the active phase of the disease.

In order to evaluate the direct impact of LKS on written language, one must also take into account the possibility that the child had a pre-existing developmental deficit preventing this type of learning, but was too young for this to be known before the epilepsy started. The children with LKS with a history of delayed language development, like those with a diagnosis of DLD (see Chapter 6) are at risk of late written language acquisition and dyslexia. Actually, a history of dyslexia is often found in families of children with LKS (Rejnö-Habte Selassie 2010). In several recent clinical studies of children with rolandic epilepsy and their siblings, difficulties with reading acquisition are often reported, probably independently from the epilepsy, but perhaps based on a common genetic background, although this is still debated (Clarke et al. 2007).

As an epileptic dysfunction can preferentially affect different subsets of networks located in the perisylvian and related regions, and this at different periods in development, one can expect to see patients with dissociated oral and written language skills. For example, oral comprehension and production can be lost (or at least for sometime) while written language is preserved or the vice versa. Not surprisingly, such cases are difficult to document and hard evidence is lacking, but there are suggestive case reports.

The most frequent situation is the expected one in which written language is affected together with oral language and whatever knowledge the child had acquired is lost. One rarely has an initial precise comparison point on the patient's level of written language before disease onset except in older children who had reached good basic mastery. Papagno and Basso (1993) reported a girl aged 8 years and 6 months who had developed moderately severe LKS (poor verbal comprehension and progressive impairment of verbal expression). She was in the third grade and learning normally. She was rapidly diagnosed and treated with adrenocorticotropic hormone (ACTH). A neuropsychological assessment of oral and written language in all its dimensions performed from the peak of the disorder at 8 years and 8 months and repeated at short intervals (8y 10m, 9y 9m,10y and 9y) allowed the team to document a rapid full recovery of oral language within 4 months. Written language however recovered only 3 months later. This precise documentation was informative because regression happened at an age when enough and good mastery was achieved. The observed course with complete and rapid recovery is probably representative of what occurs in later-onset milder cases that are rarely studied in such detail.

In earlier onset LKS, more severe or late diagnosed patients or in those who had not yet or just started to learn written language, the situation is very different and the child often never develops functional reading and writing skills. It is very difficult to know how much this is the direct result of the epileptic dysfunction, a pre-existing developmental disorder or the lack of exposure and teaching during critical periods. In addition, lack of interest and motivation can also play a role and possibly a combination of all these factors may contribute to an individual's difficulties.

There are reports of older children who had acquired written language without oral language difficulties, and whose disorder started with an isolated loss or regression of these skills before oral language became affected (Dugas et al. 1982).

The opposite, apparently exceptional situation, has also been described. A child with severe acquired VAA and almost no speech was reported by Rapin et al. (1977; Case 1, see case report and Fig 5.3): The child kept his well-developed writing and reading abilities as long as the auditory channel was by-passed.

This boy was 8 years and 6 months old when he developed VAA, loss of speech with marked fluctuations (recovery and relapses) until full and definitive return of normal language occurred at around the age of 10 years. On late follow-up in 2012, he is doing well and his daughter was diagnosed with rolandic epilepsy (I Rapin, personal communication, 2012).

During the period, he could not understand and speak, he used written language to communicate. Reading comprehension during silent reading was normal, and he could write some single letters and words to dictation, but made phonemic errors, apparently reflecting what he heard. Remarkably, he copied a word perfectly in cursive writing, whereas he wrote in print with errors to dictation, and he could read words he had been unable to write. At the age of 12, his oral reading was good except for occasional semantic paraphasias. He could understand a word spelled to him, providing it had less than six letters.

This case shows a remarkable sparing of reading and writing abilities in face of a severe oral comprehension and speech expression deficit. He could manage at school, thanks to this. Specifically, a striking difference in the motor programming of writing, that is, between fluent ability in cursive versus printed letters was demonstrated at some point. This depended whether the word was retrieved from visual versus oral language store, illustrating that a direct route from the visual written lexicon to his personal cursive graphomotor programme was intact.

There are patients with LKS with severe prolonged or even permanent auditory agnosia who develop remarkable skills in reading and writing via a purely or mainly visual route (Denes 1986; Pullens 2015). Denes et al. (1986) reported a boy who had LKS at 3 years and never recovered. At 6 years, he was taught to match objects to the corresponding written word and subsequently was able to read and write to such an extent that he could attend primary school. When tested at 11 years, his phonemic discrimination, identification and production were absent, whereas lexical-semantic abilities tested through reading and writing were normal for his age. We know of other similar remarkable unpublished cases (see Chapter 13).

In less severe cases in which phonologic representations of known words are being restored and new ones can be learned, the teaching of letters, that is, matching the visual aspect of sound to its oral counterpart, will exercise and stabilize the deficient auditory phonemic and syllabic discrimination that are crucial features for word identification. Exact sound features of a word can be repeatedly checked and confirmed/corrected and be a major support to the child. Early exposure to written language can thus facilitate both progress in oral language and in learning to read and write. Depending on the child's progression in auditory–perceptual recovery, he may first learn and enjoy having a sight visual vocabulary (logographic stage) and later uses an alphabetic strategy in reading (with a phase when both are used), a strategy that is also used by typically developing children. We are not aware of detailed longitudinal published studies of this situation in a child with LKS

Probably unique preferential routes can develop. Plaza et al. (2001) reported a child who at age of 2 years 4 months had developed comprehension difficulties and later speech loss; he was diagnosed with LKS at 3 years 4 months. He gradually improved and at 6 years, he began to read, spell and comprehend oral language and his language became more fluent. At 8 years his reading and spelling were average; he still had difficulty repeating long words, but his speech was quite fluent with good vocabulary. At 8 years and 6 months, an extensive neuropsychological examination showed that his performances on visually presented verbal memory tasks (word order, digit recall and story recall) were much better than when presented auditorily. This suggested to the authors that he had developed compensatory strategies allowing him to acquire phonologic skills from predominantly visual input.

It is likely that interesting and significant dissociations in written language competences and unusual patterns of dyslexia or closely related symbolic written representations (mathematics) will increasingly be described within the spectrum of LKS–EAS as well as unique strategies or compensatory routes that are never seen in normal development.

The variety of mechanisms that enter into written language competence and that can be either affected or spared in LKS justify opposite but equally important caveats. On the one hand, even when there is good oral language recovery, one has to suspect difficulties in written language acquisition. Attention to this aspect and early support must be given in the follow-up of the child, like that in children with a DLD or a family history of dyslexia who are at high risk in this domain. On the other hand, while a child with LKS often has prolonged or permanent written language difficulties, this should not be taken as an ineluctable fatality, even in severe cases. Children with late acquired, short lived and moderate oral language impairment may end up with normal written language learning and performances and attend mainstream school. This can also occur in children who had a prolonged period of global auditory agnosia (see Chapter 13).

One important question is whether a child with LKS can start at a very late age to learn effectively to read and write, when it was not possible or not even tried before. We have anecdotal evidence that this can happen, as is sometimes seen with developmental dyslexia, and it would be interesting to have precise longitudinal data on that.

Finally, written testimonies of adults, such as Christina and David (see Chapter 14), who had severe LKS and who, despite residual difficulties, were willing to write and talk insightfully about their experiences are an amazing source of information at a both scientific and existential level.

Cognitive and behavioural disorders in LKS: aphasia as a part of a more pervasive regression
Behavioural disorders in LKS

Major behavioural problems are frequent in LKS, either as a psychological consequence of the language impairment or as a result of the epilepsy-induced dysfunction in relevant cerebral networks (Rossi et al. 1999, Robinson et al. 2001). Both can be combined and can predominate at different times and stages of the disease.

At disease onset, a psychological cause is often considered a first explanation, and it can take time until a correct diagnosis is made. This is especially difficult when the loss of verbal comprehension is partial or intermittent, or when it occurs in a period of an unrelated family crisis in which psychological explanations for the problematic behaviour are naturally put forward.

Some children with VAA and preserved non-verbal cognitive functions can adapt sometimes surprisingly well to their language loss. They probably had naturally and culturally
well-developed non-verbal communication before disease onset. This is an impressive
experience for the clinician who first meets this situation. Such cases have contributed to
the image of 'pure' or 'typical' LKS, that is, an acquired VAA without other disabilities
and made it difficult to conceptualize that children with additional severe cognitive or
psychiatric problems could have basically the same disorder.

The combination of different acquired cognitive–behavioural disabilities besides language is multi-fold, both in nature and across the course in the disorder. The case mentioned
by Glos et al. (2001) in a report focused on a different aspect of LKS (see Fig 5.8) illustrates
this point. This child had a transient self-limited episode of major global regression ('ceased
to feed herself, incontinence, smelled toys' two years after the onset of LKS with a typical
VAA and finally a good long-term outcome. Such episodes of regression can be found in
several case histories of children with LKS (Deonna 1977).

Attention-deficit hyperactivity-disorder (ADHD) and oppositional behaviour are frequently observed at the same time or even before language impairment is recognized.
Sometimes, these behavioural disturbances can be severe; these are as much of a complaint
as the language deficit and persist long after the language deficit has recovered. Of course,
they can be the exacerbation of a pre-existing developmental ADHD, like a DLD can
precede an LKS (see discussion Chapter 6).

Sleep is often disturbed in LKS; the child has difficulty in falling asleep or/and maintaining sleep (Neville et al. 2000). It can be an early sign of the disease, which is often

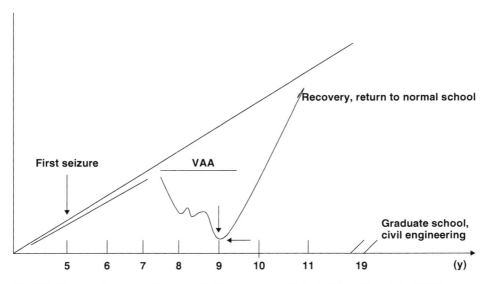

Fig. 5.8. The overall course of Landau-Kleffner syndrome. (Adapted from Glos et al., 2001.)

found in retrospect but was not much put forward because the subsequent symptoms were much more dramatic. When severe, sleep problems can obscure an incipient language impairment and can be interpreted as a psychological reaction of whatever cause and delay the diagnosis of LKS.

Children with LKS can also have unexplained episodes of fear and panic that may represent epileptic auditory hallucinations (see Chapter 5).Only after recovery and on specific questioning, sometimes much later, does one realize that the child went through such frightening experiences he was unable to share during the acute phase. There are understandably very limited data on this issue (Morrell et al. 1995; Deonna and Roulet-Perez 2005).

A mother described it in writing about her 4-year-old. 'Onset of fear without serious reason, irritation and crying close to hysteric sometimes'; 'The hysteric crises increased in frequency, it happened as if it was triggered by something, you could never expect from what; he started to scream for 15–20 minutes and then continued to behave normally as nothing happened'. When asked if that could have been auditory hallucinations, she said 'why not,' and that she 'had not thought about it'.

Some children with LKS who initially and for a prolonged time had 'only' language impairment can later present a severe attention deficit, a cognitive regression and/or psychotic behaviour, either as a new complaint or a major aggravation of the previous picture.

The many different intricate reasons that can account for behavioural disturbances in LKS are best illustrated when one sees the dramatic changes that can occur as a result of either an epilepsy-related or an environmental change. For instance, ADHD can sometimes improve with more effective antiepileptic therapy in correlation with suppression of the paroxysmal EEGs discharges. On the other hand, behaviour can improve dramatically when a substitutive means of communication is offered. It is impressive to see how the behaviour and '*joie de vivre*' of a child and his family can radically change within a short period after the introduction of sign language, sometimes after months or years of extremely limited or absent verbal understanding and speech (see Chapter 12).

COGNITIVE AND BEHAVIOURAL REGRESSION AS THE MAJOR COMPONENT OF LKS OR OBSCURING THE SPECIFIC LANGUAGE DISABILITY

Two situations have to be distinguished regarding cognitive and behavioural regression. The first is when a child with LKS develops in the course of the disorder an additional cognitive and/or severe behavioural regression that is part of the evolution of the epilepsy. The latter can be extremely severe, and the children may become unmanageable.

A striking example of such cases can be found in the study of Irwin et al. (2001) in five children who were submitted to multiple subpial transection (MST) because a severe, prolonged and drug resistant form of global aphasia. The authors insisted that 'the most striking effect was on behavior which was immediate and sustained, whereas effects on language and cognition "were less dramatic"'. All children had been either destructive or unmanageable or were regressed and withdrawn before surgery. As a mother of one of Irwin's cases told one of the authors (TD), 'as soon after he recovered from the operation, his behavior was so much improved (and has remained so) that I told myself then: even if language does not return, this will have been a major improvement'. Irwin's observations, which have probably not been given the recognition they deserve, suggests that the cessation – via MST – of the bilateral epileptic activity (CSWS were observed in all cases) that also influences the function of more remote prefrontal cortical areas (see Chapters 10 and 11) played a major role in this clinical improvement.

The second situation is that of children who present initially with a cognitive and behavioural regression, often with autistic features, and whose impaired communication and verbal language seems to be a secondary manifestation. Only when the child improves in his behaviour and when formal language testing becomes possible can one discover a specific unexpected deficit in that domain. Some data about such children can be found in series of case series of ECSWS. Debiais et al. (2007) looked at language development in a series of 10 children with ECSWS, excluding children with 'agnosia-aphasia syndrome and symptomatic CSWS'. Children had extensive specific neuropsychological and language tests, mostly done several years after onset of the syndrome (9y and 4m to 23y) in the recovery period or in the chronic residual phase (epileptic EEGs foci were still present in various locations or bilaterally). Children had weak scores in tests measuring lexical, morphosyntaxic and pragmatic skills, which could not be accounted for by their (low) cognitive level.

In our own adult follow-up study of 10 children with non-lesional ECSWS who presented initially with a cognitive–behavioural deterioration (Segmuller 2012), we also found residual language deficits unexplained by low IQ in three patients; one had a language delay before disease onset and two had a verbal regression in addition to their cognitive deterioration during the acute phase. These data indicate that within the EAS, some children can manifest either a combination or a succession of different manifestations and other language deficits beside VAA and when changes in the extent and the activity of the epilepsy occur.

In children with prefrontal epileptic foci and CSWS having phases of severe regression with apathy and lack of initiative, language production and comprehension may be altered. In this situation, impairments are not necessarily of aphasic nature but can result from severe and global executive deficits. When these improve, language appears preserved in its formal aspects, albeit its content and verbal reasoning can remain poor (Roulet-Perez et al. 1993).

Finally, there are children, within the EAS in whom very early acquired 'epileptic' cognitive–behavioural regression masquerades as a developmental disorder. This opens the much debated issue of LKS presenting with autistic features and mistaken for a developmental ASD (Deonna 2010; Stefanatos 2011). This will be discussed in Chapter 6.

6
DEVELOPMENTAL ASPECTS OF LANDAU-KLEFFNER SYNDROME/ EPILEPSY-APHASIA SPECTRUM AND THE OVERLAP WITH DEVELOPMENTAL LANGUAGE DISORDERS AND AUTISM SPECTRUM DISORDERS

The possibility that early onset of Landau-Kleffner syndrome (LKS) could be a treatable cause of language impairment in some children presenting with developmental language disorders (DLD, Bishop 2014) or autistic spectrum disorder (ASD) has been a topic of intense research in the past two decades of the twentieth century. This coincided with three simultaneous advances in different fields:

(1) Classification of epilepsies and epilepsy syndromes with the recognition of LKS as a distinct entity (Deonna and Roulet-Perez 1995a; Deonna 1999). This period also showed major developments in childhood epileptology with the discovery of new aetiologies such as cortical dysplasias with modern imaging techniques, improved electroencephalogram (EEG) monitoring with videos and new treatments, including epilepsy surgery (Roulet-Perez et al. 2010).

(2) Pioneering work in developmental neuropsychology with the definition and classification of different developmental language syndromes (Bishop and Rosenblooom 1987; Rapin 1988).

(3) Advances in research on ASD with the accurate description of the first symptoms and evolution, co-occurrence with DLD, associated neurological disturbances and search for specific aetiologies (Rapin 1991).

These advances allowed the recognition of the high rate of epilepsy in children with ASD as well as the fact that up to a third of children diagnosed with ASD had a history of regression during the second year of life, after a phase of normal or nearly normal early development (for a review of this topic, see Rapin 1995; Deonna 2010; Stefanatos 2011). Many of these new data increased the suspicion that epilepsy could account or contribute to the clinical picture.

Based on this background and a large amount of hope, many studies of children with DLD and ASD were performed, looking for evidence of subtle epileptic seizures, or 'hidden epilepsy' (i.e. epileptiform discharges without obvious clinical correlate), especially during sleep. Several studies tried to correlate the epilepsy variables with the dynamics of development (stagnation or regression, including 'autistic regression') and type of language disorders. According to the principles of evidence-based medicine, the only proof of a direct correlation between epilepsy (or epileptiform abnormalities) on the EEG and language/ behavioural impairment could only come from the demonstration of significant improvement after cessation of the epileptic activity with treatment. This however was never achieved or achieved only very rarely. Mostly, the studies were not considered proper therapeutic trials, or deemed almost impossible to interpret, given the number and complexity of the variables involved. The conclusion of all this research was that epilepsy or interictal epileptiform discharges (IEDs) were in most cases only a marker of the underlying, often genetic brain disorder, without ruling out that in exceptional cases, they could have a causal or important contributory role (Deonna et al. 1993c, 1995b).

This whole issue has somewhat fallen into disrepute, but we feel important to revisit it here.

DLD and early onset of LKS

LKS was initially described in children who had normal language for their age at the time they lost it or at least whose language development was not a concern previously. Although, most subsequently reported cases started between 3 and 7 years (an average 3-year-old masters the main linguistic dimensions of his native language), there were cases with much earlier onset. This was clear in the few diagnosed children who had an exceptionally early language development with advanced comprehension at the age of 1 and formed sentences at 18 months or 2 years and who lost these skills. In normally developing language, one can see periods of slower alternating with more rapid progress, and sometimes the apparent loss or temporary lack of use of previously mastered items (including words), while others are progressing more quickly (Bates et al. 1992). This makes it difficult to determine if a stagnation or a loss is significant and pathological unless it is marked, persistent or worsens over time (Deonna et al. 1982). The rapid normal pace of development of a given function can initially mask a slowly interfering pathological until regression becomes evident as seen in some neurodegenerative diseases. In addition, fluctuations in language development can occur for different reasons, in this age group typically intermittent hypoacousis from glue-ears.

Consequently, in the younger subgroup of children finally diagnosed with LKS, the dynamics of early language development is most often unclear. Data on the quality and quantity of language attained and on its developmental pace (rapid or slow) at disease onset are rare. Questions such as 'Was the child in a slow or more rapid phase of language acquisition when the epileptic activity started?' and 'What dimension of language was mainly affected?' are often not asked.

In all reported cases of LKS (usually several years later), many had 'normal language development' without further details; some had a slightly delayed language development, not severe enough to require a specialist's attention. However, a few of them had a previous speech and language evaluation and therapy or had been formally diagnosed with a DLD. These were usually making progress when the regression set in. Stefanatos et al. (2002), in a literature review of 208 cases found that about 10% of all cases of LKS had started at or before the age of 2 (i.e. the age when a regression of language was reported), but details on the type and severity of the initial impairments were not available (or not looked for) in these children.

There are a few exceptions we know of. One of our patients was seen by a speech therapist at the age of 5 years and 6 months for an isolated articulation disorder (case GA, Chapter 5). An audio-recorded full language examination was obtained and reviewed by us, confirming this finding. Six months later, he presented with comprehension difficulties and a speech regression. Another child we heard of (G Offermanns, personal communication, 2015) had late language development and a first formal language assessment at the age of 4. Production was poor, but receptive phonology was within normal limits. One year later, he had made progress in expressive phonology, but had not normalized, and he was diagnosed with a DLD at the age of 6. Within the following year, he regressed, mainly in language comprehension and a diagnosis of LKS was made. This case is important, because of a documented expressive language disorder at the age of 4 with no comprehension deficit and progresses until his 7th year when a deficit in this latter domain appeared. This course suggests a pre-existing developmental expressive language disorder with a later acquired receptive deficit. In cases like these, the initial language delay is likely to be a genetically determined developmental disorder, affecting language networks, related or not to the subsequent LKS (separate familial DLD or shared genetic cause of DLD and focal epilepsy; see Chapter 9; also see Turner [2015] on genes involved in language and epilepsy). There is no good argument in these cases to attribute the DLD to the later found epileptic activity, albeit no EEG was performed before the regression occurred.

The course of language development in children with early onset of LKS, that is, before the age of 18–24 months, is schematized in Figure 6.1. When no stagnation or regression can be documented (see Figure 6.1c) but only slow development, the diagnosis rests on the EEG findings and clear correlative improvement with antiepileptic therapy (see discussion below on DLD and epileptiform discharges).

There are documented cases with early onset and recovery under therapy. The child reported by Uldall et al. (2000) is one of the few with a correlative language/EEG/ therapy follow-up study that also well illustrates the diagnostic, therapeutic and assessment challenges. This boy 'lost acquired language and became mute' within 3 to 6 months following a probable seizure at 18 months (he had already suffered a single febrile seizure at 11mo). A 'pervasive developmental disorder or developmental dysphasia' was suspected by a child psychiatrist. A diagnosis of LKS was made 1 year and 6 months later (at 3y 3mo). There was moderate improvement with clobazam and vigabatrin. Prednisone was started 1 year and 6 months later (4y 9mo) and for only 2 ½ months due to the parent's reluctance. A dramatic improvement was seen, with a yearly increase in active vocabulary within 3 months. He slowly progressed, but plateaued at the age of 6. A second course of prednisone had a similar positive effect: He 'improved his comprehension and vocabulary almost to a normal level'.

Importantly, but not emphasized in the abstract (although fully discussed by the authors) speech production was more affected than comprehension across the whole course and the child did not seem to have verbal auditory agnosia (VAA) at any point. He also had a normal first EEG, including sleep at 18 months, and from the age of 33 months bitemporal paroxysms, 'typical of LKS'. He never had CSWS (12 sleep tracings).

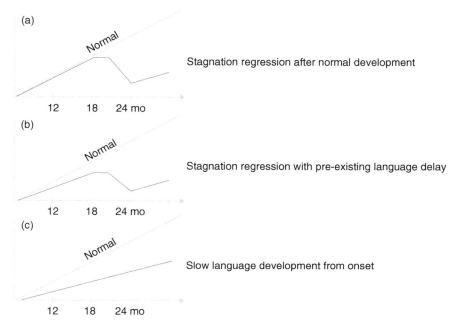

Fig. 6.1. Language development, stagnation-regression in cases of Landau-Kleffner syndrome with early onset.

A follow-up was given to TD by the author (P Uldall, personal communication 2012). At the age of 11, the child's verbal IQ was 68 and performance IQ 101 on Wechsler Scale. On the last follow-up at the age of 18, he just managed to pass an exam at the ninth-grade level. He reports expressive difficulties when he is stressed.

EPILEPTIFORM DISCHARGES IN DLD: MARKER OR CAUSE?

The first systematic approach to find out whether and which children diagnosed with DLD could actually have an early form of LKS was to look for focal epileptiform abnormalities, especially sleep-activated focal spikes or sharp waves or diffuse IEDs on the EEG. Depending on the inclusion criteria of the cohort – children with or without history of seizures, severity of language impairment, including receptive deficits and referral bias, that is, hospital versus community-based – a variable percentage ranging from 10% to 50% of children were found to have epileptiform discharges or more specifically FSW (Maccario et al. 1982; Echenne 1990, 1998; Echenne et al. 1992; Duvelleroy-Hommet et al. 1995; Parry-Fielder et al. 1997, 2009; Picard et al. 1998; Neuschlová et al. 2007; Billard et al. 2009; Rejnö-Habte Selassie 2010). The final and only robust conclusion of these studies was that in children with a DLD (defined as isolated language impairment without associated deficits), epilepsy or IEDs were neither causal nor a contributing factor. Exceptions to this statement and the indication for an EEG in DLD are discussed at the end of this chapter.

The few studies in which a trial with antiepileptic drugs was attempted in children who had language impairments and IEDs gave negative or unconvincing results (Picard et al. 1998; Billard et al. 2009).

Without a strict longitudinal follow-up with correlative clinical/EEG documentation, it is actually difficult to demonstrate a definite drug-induced benefit, except in rare spectacular cases.

Two examples of children we had the opportunity to meet early on and in whom a clinical-linguistic neuropsychological and correlative EEG follow-up was possible are given below.

Speech delay due to a pre-linguistic regression of epileptic origin
Julian 26-month-old boy, was seen in our outpatient clinic for recent onset of seizures during sleep. His EEG showed bilateral mainly right-sided asynchronous centrotemporal focal sharp waves compatible with an early-onset rolandic epilepsy. Brain MRI was normal. He had at this time an isolated severe speech delay with only rare vocalizations and single syllables. A retrospective analysis of family videos of his productions from the babbling stage at the age of 8 months to 26 months and a prospective study from 28 to 50 months (measuring the repertoire of consonants and number of utterances/min) were performed. It revealed a normal early babbling stage from 8 to 12 months, but a qualitative and quantitative regression of his productions form 12 to 15 months. After a long stagnation, a rapid increase of productions was observed after 26 months when the seizures stopped and the EEG normalized. At the age of 4, his speech and language were normal. In retrospect nocturnal seizures probably started before the age of 12 months with spontaneous phases of remissions and relapses. This longitudinal study shows that what was interpreted as a developmental speech delay was in fact the result of an early regression of emergent pre-linguistic skills due to a focal, probably bilateral epileptic dysfunction (Mayor Dubois et al. 2004).

Early acquired versus congenital verbal auditory agnosia with focal EEG abnormalities and spontaneous recovery (Mayor, Roulet-Perez, Deonna, unpublished)
Kevin was first seen at the age of 2 years 9 months for absence of expressive and receptive language and behavioural difficulties. His non-verbal performances were borderline normal (Bailey scale 70–76). Seizures were never reported. Brainstem auditory evoked potential was normal. Loss of emerging verbal productions was in retrospect suspected between ages 1 and 2, but could not be firmly established despite direct contact with his paediatrician and visits to the family. A first EEG at 2 years 9 months showed intermittent left central focal sharp waves activated by sleep. We decided not to introduce immediate therapy, because there was doubt about regression and because the EEG abnormalities were unilateral and not sustained. Integration in a kindergarten for deaf children was immediately proposed. He rapidly learned signs with a deaf adult in school. Behaviour improved rapidly as soon as he could communicate, which he did exclusively in sign language for about 6 months. Oral language started between 3 and 4 years with unexpected quick improvement. A second EEG (waking and sleep) at 3 years 6 months was normal. At 4 years 9 months, formal language tests showed nearly normal comprehension, a lexical level of 3 years and 6 months and a phonological-syntactic level at the 2 years and 6 months, with a sentence production up to five words. At 6 years, he was following normal elementary school with speech therapy (Fig 6.2).

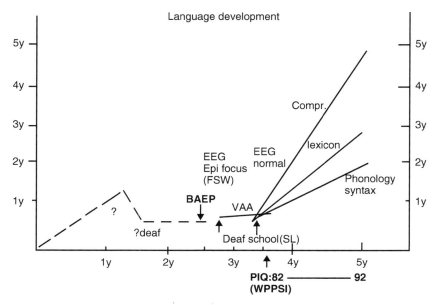

Fig. 6.2. Early acquired versus congenital verbal auditory agnosia with focal EEG abnormalities and spontaneous recovery Compr., comprehension; FSW, focal spike waves; BAEP, brainstem auditory evoked potentials; VAA, verbal auditory agnosia; SL, sign language; WPPSI, Wechsler Preschool and Primary Scale of Intelligence.

It remains uncertain whether this child's initial paroxysmal EEG abnormalities were causally related to his language deficit, which spontaneously and rapidly improved. These may have been more sustained previously and already spontaneously remitted when first recorded. The recorded IEDs may have been bilateral and more sustained before the first recording and may have caused an early language regression – that is, an early acquired epileptic VAA-and already spontaneously remitted when first recorded. On the other hand, as discussed in Chapter 8, a pre-existing network abnormality may have provided the basis for a severe receptive developmental VAA and transient epileptiform discharges. This case well illustrates the difficulty of the differential diagnosis between a severe receptive developmental versus early acquired epileptic VAA. The quick and full recovery is in favour of the latter because a severe developmental receptive language impairment usually takes years to improve and recovery is often far from complete. This is why K's documented course seems different (we have never read of such an observation) and could result from an epileptic dysfunction. In this regard, Dorothy Bishops' comment in her book *Uncommon Understanding in Children* (1997) is worth to quote:

In my early studies of children with DLD, I encountered children with the diagnosis of "receptive aphasia", where the history of regression was suggestive of LKS, but where the child never had seizures and recording had not been taken around the time of onset, so the diagnosis could not be confirmed. It would be misleading to give the impression that all children with severe receptive impairments have an epileptic aetiology (whether recognized or undiagnosed). However, in my experience, those rare children who seem able to make little sense of sound despite having adequate hearing and normal development in other respects, do not seem to be on a continuum with other types of developmental language disorders, at least as far as aetiology is concerned, and it seems prudent to study them as a separate group until we have stronger justification for treating them as simply a severe variant of DLD....

Both the above-reported cases open the possibility that a temporary arrest or regression in language development could be related to self-limited focal epileptic activity. This reasoning may apply to other developmental disorders such as ASD in which unexpected rapid recovery sometime takes place (see below).

INDICATIONS FOR AN EEG IN A CHILD WITH A DLD

There is now sufficient information on the long-term follow-up and low incidence of epileptiform discharges on the EEG in children with an isolated speech delay or a 'regular' DLD to discard a possible causal role of a 'hidden' epilepsy. In such cases, an EEG assessment is unnecessary. It is however indicated together with other investigations in children with a regression or stagnation of language after a normal onset and progression, a personal or family history of seizures and additional developmental problems (behaviour, motor and cognition). Regarding the type of language deficit, that is, the presence of receptive rather than expressive difficulties, especially if there is suspicion of VAA can be also an important argument. However, one has to remember here that some children later diagnosed with LKS presented with an expressive language deficit with preserved comprehension; therefore, an EEG with a sleep record is recommended in children with an unusual dysfluency, for instance, an atypical stuttering, unexplained mutism, speech dyspraxia and oromotor difficulties, especially when fluctuating or acquired.

Language and/or autistic regression

During the 30-year period discussed at the beginning of this chapter, the devastating impact of various early onset lesional epilepsies on cognitive development and behaviour became better appreciated. This was also in part supported by the results of epilepsy surgery performed at an increasingly younger age. Well-documented cases of 'acquired epileptic autistic symptoms' that were reversible with effective antiepileptic therapy were published (Roulet-Perez and Deonna 2006). It was then advocated that a sleep EEG be performed in children with an ASD to rule out epilepsy as a possible cause, even in the absence of seizures. Epileptiform discharges were frequently found on the EEG in this population, although there was no striking difference between those children who had an early 'autistic regression' and those who had not (Tuchman et al. 1991; Rapin 1995; Tuchman and Rapin 1997; McVicar et al. 2005; Baird et al. 2006).

Antiepileptic therapy was nevertheless tried in a few studies with alleged positive results (Neville et al. 1997, Nass et al. 1998, 1999a, b; Lewine et al. 1999). These studies were considered insufficiently documented, so that the possible causal role of IEDs was gradually dismissed. Seizures and IEDs are now considered an epiphenomenon of the many possible underlying brain pathologies responsible for ASDs and associated intellectual disability. A growing amount of genetic and metabolic diseases affecting molecular pathways important for brain development and neuronal excitability are identified via next generation sequencing of DNA and sophisticated metabolic analysis.

Having said that, it is important to review the rarely reported children initially diagnosed with a developmental ASD of unknown but probably genetic origin in whom a later diagnosis of LKS was made (Stefanatos et al. 2002; Deonna and Roulet-Perez 2010). The first question is whether their autistic symptoms differed from developmental ASD, either in their nature or in their course. The case reports suggest that lack of verbal communication, withdrawal and stereotypies were the main symptoms. Lack of symbolic play or understanding of social situations did not seem to be the key features in these early LKS. Some autistic behaviours in children with LKS can be attributed to a psychological reaction to the severe language deficit, both expressive and receptive, but an extension of the epileptic dysfunction to neural circuits belonging to the 'social brain' networks is also possible in some cases. A pre-existing developmental ASD must also be considered, by analogy with children who present a DLD before LKS sets in.

The pattern of onset and disappearance of the autistic symptoms in correlation with the control of the epileptic activity in these early LKS children could be interesting to observe in this respect. Will the different components of the autistic triad (impairment in communication, social interaction and restricted interests and repertoire of behaviours) appear or improve at the same or at a different pace? If, for instance, the language impairment improves first, then this could indicate its weight compared to other autistic behaviours, whether the different components of the ASD are independent or influence each other (see 'Eloise's case in Chapter 14).

In their retrospective follow-up study of 19 children with LKS (Rejnö-Habte Selassie et al. 2010), some among them had early onset epilepsy, two had a previous diagnosis of ASD, one of 'atypical autism' and three had a milder social dysfunction (based on the Asperger syndrome screening questionaire). However, the authors did not specify whether the reported autistic features had always been present or were acquired or aggravated during the course of their epilepsy.

We did not find any report of a child whose clinical picture was that of a 'pure' ASD with preserved non-verbal intelligence who later recovered, either spontaneously or with treatment from an idiopathic focal epilepsy with abundant sleep-activated IEDs. The reported children always had autistic features in combination with language, cognitive and sometimes motor impairments, with or without a history of regression or plateauing. They had either seizures or only sleep-activated focal/multifocal IEDs sometimes meeting the criteria of CSWS. Some improved markedly with AED therapy and 'lost' their autistic behaviours (Zappella 2010; Canitano 2006). Unfortunately, the additional cognitive and behavioural disturbances in most of these children rendered a formal longitudinal study of the different components of the clinical picture and their respective response to therapy very difficult to disentangle.

Children diagnosed with ASD (usually between ages 3 and 4) whose history reveals an early language and autistic regression (before the age of 2y to 2y 6mo) are usually studied months or years after the onset of the deterioration. It is, therefore, almost impossible to know whether the language regression can sometimes occur independently from and precede the regression in social interaction. Reports by child psychiatrists who interviewed parents of the children who regressed suggest that the loss of verbal and social-communicative skills is simultaneous. The children's previous vocabulary seems to have been limited to 'not more than 10 words', which they called 'reflex words', meaning that they were produced in a specific context or in response to the same stimulus ('stimulus response pairs') (Frith et al. 2003 in Novartis Symp, 2003). Of course, these children were considered to have 'idiopathic' developmental ASD and were not investigated for an underlying epileptic aetiology, neither during the acute phase nor later.

To our knowledge, there is only one case report suggesting that an early regression in verbal language can occur before a regression in social interaction as a result of an epileptic dysfunction (Chilosi et al. 2014).

In this longitudinal observational study (Chilosi et al. 2014), this boy presented with two episodes of regression at 25 and 36 months of age without seizures. He had focal IEDs and both behaviour and EEG markedly improved with ACTH therapy. After analyzing and correlating the retrospective study of the family videos from the age of 16 months, the results of language and other questionnaires and the direct observations by professionals since he was first seen at 25 months, it was possible to establish that the initial regression affected language comprehension and expression a few months before social interaction and communication. This study showed that, despite its limitations, the conditions for approaching such a complex issue can be met in exceptional circumstances, when the different specialists involved collaborate and adequate tools such as questionnaires on early language development and autistic behavior as well as serial video recordings of the child in different settings are available (Chilosi et al. 2014).

Twins or siblings with EAS syndromes and cognitive–behavioural impairments but discordant profiles

The observations of siblings or twins having a similar focal epilepsy syndrome in the EAS spectrum but presenting discordant clinical profiles of developmental or acquired disability have not been sufficiently put forward.

For instance, one twin can have an acquired aphasia and the other a DLD (Rapin et al. 1977; Echenne et al. 1992; Deonna and Roulet-Perez 2005; Praline et al. 2006). A remarkable family was reported by Roubertie et al. (2003) presenting different profiles of developmental and acquired cognitive impairments associated with sleep-activated IEDs and no visible lesion on brain MRI: patient one, a boy from a dizygous twin pair had the most severe phenotype with global developmental delay, subsequently worsened by an autistic regression. He had epileptic seizures and his EEGs showed bifrontal spike waves with CSWS. Their variation in density coincided with phases of regression and improvements. His co-twin, a girl, had a DLD of a phonologic-syntactic type and an attention deficit but normal intellect. She neither had seizures nor episodes of regression. An older sister had isolated moderate IED and no seizures either. The EEG of both girls showed bilateral mildly sleep-activated focal IEDs. In this family, cognitive impairments and IED are very likely to be due to a common genetic factor. Phenotypic variability may be attributed to variable expression of the genetic trait in different but closely related cognitive networks, by other unknown modifying genes or environmental factors. However, as in the family with auto-somic dominant rolandic epilepsy and speech dyspraxia (ADRESD; see Chapter 8 and 9) identified as having a mutation in *GRIN2A* and in another family with a *GRIN2A* mutation (family D in Carvill 2013), the intense sleep-activated IEDs have certainly contributed to phases of regression and worsening of the baseline phenotype.

Conclusion

In order to explain ASD, impaired neuronal connectivity throughout the whole brain has been hypothesized for a long time. Recently, however, novel functional imaging techniques applied to specific cohorts of patients with autism tend to show that networks constituting the 'social brain' (including among others structures such as orbito-, medio- and prefrontal cortex, temporo-parietal junction and amygdala) are more specifically involved (Frith and Frith 2007; Adolph 2009; Lahnakoski et al. 2012). For instance, in a recent study of high-functioning adolescents with an ASD via a whole brain connectivity fMRI (Gotts et al. 2012), the authors concluded that 'not only are decreases in connectivity most pronounced between regions of the social brain but also that they are selective to connections between limbic-related regions involved in affective aspects of social processes from other parts of the brain that support language and sensory motor processing'. An important 'hub' for social cognition is the posterior part of the superior temporal sulcus receiving visual and auditory information (Lahnakoski 2012) and is particularly relevant because of its anatomi-cal closeness with the epileptogenic zone of EAS. By analogy with the previously discussed case of early rolandic epilepsy interfering with emerging expressive speech (see Julian, p. 63), one can postulate that early epileptic activity involving the posterior superior tem-poral sulcus may affect social cognition, for instance, visual recognition of facial emotions (Lepännen 2009).

7
EVOLUTION OF LANDAU–KLEFFNER SYNDROME: SHORT-, MID- AND LONG-TERM OUTCOMES

Introduction

Most neurological conditions have a spectrum of severity with the most severe cases having being identified and reported long before milder forms are recognized. This was also the case for Landau–Kleffner syndrome (LKS) for several reasons:

(1) The multiple manifestations of the disorder have been a concern for different professionals, each describing the most salient aspects of the disease at various times in its evolution.
(2) The natural history of LKS has probably been influenced negatively in the early cases by the use of classic antiepileptic drugs (carbamazepine, phenobarbital and phenytoin) that can aggravate IEDs.
(3) The narrow definition of LKS has tended to disregard cases not having verbal auditory agnosia (VAA) or milder language impairments.

The age at onset, quality and amount of language at the time of disease onset and the severity and duration of the epileptic dysfunction are of major importance for the ultimate prognosis. The severity of the language impairment and associated cognitive and behavioural disorders reflect the extent of the epilepsy-related dysfunction in the perisylvian and various connected networks. These variables are now better appreciated, thanks to diverse functional imaging tools (see Chapters 10 and 11).

Psychological dimensions such as the capacity to pay attention to spoken language after it has not made sense for a prolonged period, and the motivation to communicate again with spoken language when the disorder subsides, are also crucial for prognosis but hard to predict in individual cases.

Figure 7.1 attempts to summarize the major epilepsy-related variables that will determine the final prognosis in an individual case and that can be important at different moments of an often prolonged evolution. Dashed areas represent the predominantly involved cortical regions, either by the focal or distant effects of the epileptic activity. The perisylvian region predominantly affected in epilepsy-aphasia spectrum and prefrontal regions are indicated with their corresponding deficits. Sleep-induced activation and bilateral propagation of the

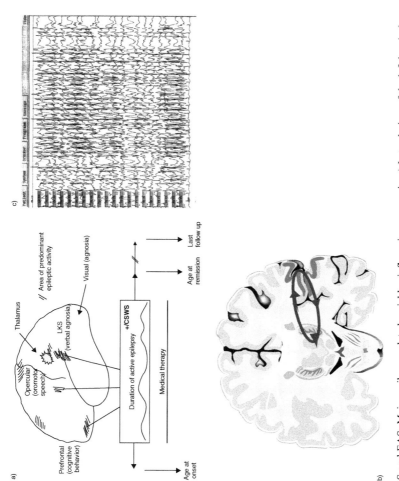

Fig. 7.1. Outcome of LKS and EAS. Major epilepsy-related variables influencing prognosis. a) Lateral view of the left hemisphere with predominant sites of epileptic activity seen in the anterior region in AEOS (acquired epileptic opercular syndrome) and posterior temporal region in LKS. The prefrontal regions are rarely the primary site of epileptic activity (LKS variants with multiple foci), but more often a site of bilateral propagation or possibly remote inhibition (see Chapter 11). Other cortical areas (such as the visual cortex) are rarely if ever the primary site. In addition to localization and propagation, age at onset, duration of the epileptiform activity and medical treatment are important parameters. b) Coronal view of the brain at the level of the thalamus showing the corticothalamic interactions. In the EAS syndromes, sleep induces an activation and bilateral propagation of the focal cortical epileptic discharges via distinct thalamo cortical circuits. This can be recorded on the surface (scalp) electroencephalogram (EEG). c) Sleep induced high amplitude diffuse CSWS (continuous spikes and waves during sleep) recorded on the scalp EEG. (de Tiège et al. 2013; see also Chapters 10 and 11).

71

Box 1: Long-term outcome of Landau-Kleffner Syndrome

Clinical

Extremes: from full to no recovery

Residual deficits in cases with +/– full recovery

      Phonological short-term memory deficit

      Difficulties with rapid processing, environmental noises

Special investigations

      Extinction dichotic listening

      Functional imaging (differences from controls)

---

focal interictal discharges (CSWS) via thalamocortical circuits contribute to the final neuropsychological outcome (deTiège et al. 2013; Galer 2014; see Chapters 10 and 11).

Outcome of the original and early recognized series of cases (1980–1990)

The review of 45 cases by Bishop (1985) and our own adult follow-up study (1989) of the cases we first published of children in 1977 showed many patients with severe sequelae. However, the follow-up data from the original series of Landau and Kleffner (Mantovani and Landau 1980) and from Kaga (1999) indicate that some made significant recovery: These four patients born in the 1960–1970s (onset respectively at 4y 3mo, 5y, 6y 4mo and 4y 7mo; 2 out of 4 with seizures 'controlled by anticonvulsants easily', no other data on therapy) were seen again at 27, 30, 28 and 34 years, respectively, and improved markedly despite a prolonged period of VAA. The most recent case series from the National Epilepsy Center in Norway of 19 children seen between 1989 and 2010 (11 followed for more than 10 years) found unsurprisingly 'that late onset of the aphasia, short duration of the initial aphasic period and marked fluctuations in speech abilities appeared to be associated with a positive outcome' (Cockerell et al. 2011).

It is difficult to conclude about clinical-electroencephalogram (EEG) correlations in the early reported cases because EEG follow-up examinations were not considered indispensible (especially with a sleep record) and were not a routine part of the follow-up of the disease. In some reports, one can suspect that a decrease in the epileptic activity on the EEG was not sufficient or did not last long enough to allow significant progress to manifest before a relapse occurred.

While it must be stressed that generalizations about prognosis in LKS are unwarranted, detailed reports on long-term outcome (see Box 1) and some more recent follow-up studies highlight important facts summarized below:

- Cases with only a 'brief' period of VAA (weeks or months) can recover fully in all respects, including written language.
- Cases with severe global VAA of some duration (1–2 years) can also have a good if not full (complete) recovery with mild sequelae.
- Some cases with long-standing auditory agnosia of several years duration still can have a late substantial recovery of verbal comprehension and expressive speech (Vance 1991; Zardini et al. 1995; Roulet-Perez et al. 2001, Deonna et al. 2009; Downes et al. 2015).

This outcome was not thought possible previously, but has been well documented. Remediation focussing on retraining auditory attention and speech discrimination permitted remarkable improvement in some cases (see Chapter 13).

• Cases with global and permanent auditory agnosia seem to be now extremely rare, but even nowadays, many experienced clinicians have kept in mind a child who made no significant language recovery, despite the disappearance of seizures and IEDs.

Modes of recovery

Precise correlative longitudinal therapeutic/EEG studies are necessary to show that therapy actually modifies the natural course of the disorder. To better understand how the epileptic activity and possibly other factors interfere with language and cognition in LKS, it is important to document not only that language recovery takes place but also the dynamics and the order of recovery of the various language components. There are very few such studies and curiously for opposite reasons. When recovery is rapid and obvious, no special effort is made to document how it occurred. When protracted, many intervening events may complicate the assessment, and there is little motivation for studying what appear insignificant changes.

RAPID RESTORATION OF 'NORMAL' COMPREHENSION AND/OR EXPRESSION

In this situation, the epileptic dysfunction in the language networks has subsided, and their organization has apparently been unaltered. This is more likely to occur when there is a short active epilepsy course, a later onset (when the networks are already stabilized), predominant unilateral IEDs and of course early effective therapy. One would expect that well-automatized language skills – that is, early acquired and thus more stable and 'hard-wired' – will recover before the more recently acquired ones, for instance, recovery of oral before written language or recovery of a first before a second language. An example of the latter is given by a case of Korff and Deonna (unpublished): this multi-lingual boy (four languages!) experienced steroid sensitive short recurrent episodes of VAA from the age of 5 (see case report in Chapter 12 p. 132). The child first improved in Russian (his mother tongue) then in English (spoken in elementary school), then Arabic (his father's tongue) and finally French (his babysitter's and living place language), according to length and perhaps amount of exposure to each language. Bishop (1982) mentioned that in two boys she observed, 'in both cases, the child had well developed language skills with a distinctive regional accent prior to onset. Despite the fact that these children attended residential schools far from their home-town, as their language recovered, they spoke again with the original accent, which was quite unlike that used by their teachers. It seems that these children do not need to relearn language, but that their recovery involves restoration of preexisting skills', p. 710. This is congruent with the fact that prosody (that accounts for regional accent) has an early onset in normal development, before pronunciation of words is fully mastered (see Chapter 5).

SLOW, PROGRESSIVE RESTORATION OF LANGUAGE

When the deficit has been long lasting, a complete or partial disruption of networks that support a given language component, for instance, phonological representations or lexical storage, may have occurred. In this situation, the skill must be learned anew.

Table 7.1 Recovery of speech process over 2 years

6 years (March 2002)	6 year 5 months (October 2002)	8 years (March 2004)
E sisissisiEpEpEpEC pourquoi des caractères différents ? traduction en bas?	E Un ga.. on et un fill i jouent ballon C	E le gar on il est triste parce que la grenouille.elle n'est plus ici

An example of slow but full recovery of language in a child (Claude) with severe VAA and almost complete loss of speech was documented in one of our cases, (Mayor-Dubois, unpublished). Table 7.1 shows the verbal description of the same image story (story-telling speech samples from the image booklet 'Frog, where are you', from the Mercer Mayer series of children's books) at 6 years, 6 year 5 months and 8 years and illustrates the striking recovery process of speech over a 2-year period.

Recovery started with only production of phonemes or repetitive identical syllables followed 5 months later by almost full words, mainly nouns with few grammatical and function words. Marked improvement in word content and grammar, but still incomplete words and sentences were seen 1 year and 6 months later (8 years). At 9 years, speech comprehension and production were fully normal.

Another child, aged 6 years and 6 months, with a longer duration of global aphasia before the successful effect of steroids, started to 'speak' incessantly with a jargon made of simple previously over-learned words, long repetition of syllables, without significant change in verbal comprehension. We postulated that the functional inhibition of the networks implicated in the execution of elementary syllable-word productions was alleviated first. The first utterances seem to issue from an again available preserved automatized repertoire, despite lack of receptive abilities that improved later. Another possibility was that some speech–sound perception started to recover but escaped our testing.

These patterns of productions in the early recovery phase of severe LKS with prolonged VAA and speech loss that emerged after suppression of IEDs by drugs are quite striking. They neither resemble productions of typically developing children learning to speak nor those of children recovering from acquired aphasia after an acute brain lesion and are possibly unique to VAA in LKS. It is likely that a variety of yet unreported and unique patterns of productions can occur during one or the other phase of the disorder in children with LKS (Chevrie-Muller et al. 1991).

RAPID THEN SLOW (OR VICE-VERSA) RECOVERY IN THE SAME CHILD AT DIFFERENT PHASES OF LKS

A same child may first have a moderate and rapidly resolving deficit and later a more severe relapse with a protracted course and incomplete recovery. Inversely, a child with a prolonged and incomplete but significant recovery can relapse (sometimes during drug withdrawal) but at this time has a rapid return to the previous improved level (see Chapter 5).

Residual verbal attentional and other cognitive deficits in children with LKS

Rejnö-Habte Selassié et al. (2010) carried what is probably the most detailed neuropsychological long-term study of children with LKS, because it also included the assessment of other cognitive functions besides language. The 19 children of the study were representative of the different ages at onset and dynamics of the language impairment before diagnosis and were classified as follows:

(1) Normal initial language development and later stagnation/regression of language labelled 'definite LKS' (six patients).
(2) Delayed initial language development and subsequent stagnation/regression labelled 'probable LKS' (three patients).
(3) Late initial language development followed by persistent slow language development labelled 'possible LKS'.

The children classified as 3 were also called 'epileptic language disorder' (10 children). Detailed information on the seizure history, EEG findings (including sleep), brain imaging and family history (positive in >50% for seizure disorder and/or cognitive difficulties) clearly showed that these patients belonged to the EAS spectrum and did not include cases with lesional epilepsy.

Eight patients were young adults (19–25y), and 11 were schoolchildren (8–14y) at follow-up. The findings of normal results on several speech and language parameters in 25%–50% of the cohort sample are noteworthy (Fig 7.2). Of importance is also that all patients had an auditory attention deficit demonstrated with a dichotic listening task using a forced choice paradigm and 12 out of 19 (63%) had comprehension difficulties in noisy environment.

Severe cases with limited or absent recovery
Children with this dismal outcome are mainly historical (see Chapter 13): they had severe aphasia to begin with, usually of early onset and often a delayed diagnosis, late effective therapy or refractory epilepsy with either persistence of seizures and/or active IEDs.

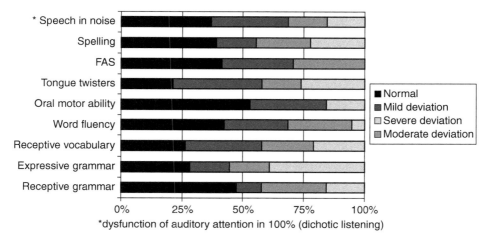

Fig. 7.2. Speech, language and auditory perception at follow-up in 19 individuals with focal epileptiform activity and language disorder in childhood. FAS, phonological word retrieval test. Reprinted from Epilepsy Behav, Rejno-Habte Selassie et al. © 2010 with permission from Elsevier.

Language networks appear to have become completely unfunctional, without possible compensation via intra- or inter-hemispheric relocation.

The more recent case series of middle- and long-term follow-up studies of LKS (Cockerell et al. 2011, 19 children; Caraballo et al. 2014, 29 children) that included children diagnosed and treated earlier and more aggressively than previously suggest that there was no severe case without speech and verbal comprehension, although no sufficient details are provided to be certain. In their retrospective review of 35 patients with severe LKS and non-lesional ECSWS who underwent pre-surgical evaluation for possible MST in the temporal lobe (see Chapter 12), Downes et al. (2015) found that 29 out of 35 patients had profound to severe language impairments at assessment and that 22 out of 25 remained so at follow-up at a mean age of 13 years. Patients were included from 1992 to 2010, showing that patients with severe LKS who already benefitted from modern therapy still exist nowadays, albeit possibly less frequently than previously. Progress in anatomic and functional brain imaging and the discovery of new genetic mutations may contribute to explain the outcome of these patients.

The question whether and how some late restoration of function can occur later in adolescence or even in adulthood, is still left unanswered. As mentioned in the introduction, the possibility of an additional 'disuse' component must be considered. Such children may have 'learned' not to pay attention to irrelevant and distorted auditory information. A few children, who had become fluent signers and did not rely on auditory information, have actually recovered functional language, thanks to intense auditory retraining (see Chapter 13 and case David in Chapter 14). How late in life such a restoration of oral language can be obtained remains to be established. A proposal for such a work in an 18-year-old girl educated with the deaf but who was recovering some auditory discrimination and used some verbal cues in daily life has unfortunately failed (case Alice, Chapter 14).

The fate of children with prolonged or permanent VAA followed for many years is described in Chapter 13.

Outcome of children with prolonged isolated speech production deficits
There are very few reports of long-term detailed clinical follow-up of patients with LKS and purely expressive aphasia or of AEOS who were speechless for prolonged periods. This makes one wonder if they in fact recover better or more completely. A child with AEOS and severe oromotor dysfunction and dysarthria from age 7–8 had fully recovered at the age of 16 (Tohyama 2011; see Chapter 7 for details). A lesser susceptibility to epilepsy-induced damage of these much earlier and more rapidly maturing networks, or a better take-over by the controlateral side could be explanations for such a good outcome. However, permanent oromotor or speech impairment can be found in severe or early onset cases of acquired epileptic opercular syndrome. These variably severe deficits are probably much less incapacitating, because a dysfunction in the motor speech network has lesser downstream effect on language than a dysfunction involving comprehension. Oromotor deficits with a component of dysarthria and verbal apraxia can be found in families reported as autosomic dominant rolandic epilepsy and speech dyspraxia (ADRESD, Sheffer 1995; Prats et al. 1999; Turner et al. 2015a, b on GRIN2A). Part of these deficits was probably already present before the epileptic activity started and was likely to be aggravated by it (see Chapters 6, 8 and 9).

The notion of full recovery

There is a big difference between marked and full recovery of language. This depends on how much language is put to the test in real life. Slow processing of verbal information when listening to a fast speaking interlocutor, presence of background noise and word finding difficulties in a narration can all be found, like in children with a developmental language disorder (DLD) who have apparently completely recovered (Bishop 1997). This is what Christine, a 28-year-old Norwegian woman, married with two children, wrote to the Oslo University Hospital, National Centre for Rare Epilepsy Related Disorders, Norway (Cockerell 2012), where she had been treated as a child for early onset of LKS (2y 5mo) and who was considered to have fully recovered:

> I wish I could talk to someone who actually knows what LKS is, and what repercussions you can get. Because there will be repercussions, and when growing up, all I wanted was to be like everybody else. Now I'm tired of reaching for the stars when I can't even reach the tree tops. Others see me as someone who functions normally, they don't realize the problem. People know what aphasia is, they picture some grandparents with speech problems. It's almost like talking about that imaginary friend from childhood that only you could see, therefore I don't talk about it – I've tried (Christine).

Several studies have shown evidence of persistent focal residual brain dysfunction in these patients using various sensitive techniques, including dichotic listening and functional brain imaging (Metz-Lutz et al. 1997, 2001; Majerus et al. 2003), even in the few adult patients who had normal results on language tests and no clinical complaints. Auditory attention and short-term verbal memory deficits can be uncovered in such adults and these may represent a significant disability in some professions with verbally and auditorily demanding conditions. These findings suggest that the persistent focal IEDs have permanently modified part of the language networks or have occurred in an already maldeveloped circuit (see Chapter 10). Written language skills that may be affected despite fully recovered oral language is an issue that has been already discussed separately (see Chapter 5) Musical abilities, apparently always affected in severe cases, are only starting to be formally assessed (Levêque et al. in preparation; also see Chapter 5 on musical abilities and Christine's story in Chapter-14).

Outcome of children with early onset/developmental LKS

One could expect that children with very early onset who can present like children with a DLD (see Chapter 6) will have a more severe long-term outcome. There has been very few if any long-term study of such children. The above-discussed Rejnö-Habte Selassie et al.'s study is an exception: 10 children without language regression but only slow development and stagnation (but otherwise similar in terms of seizures and EEG findings to those with deterioration) had no worse outcome than those who presented later with a regression. One cannot rule out that some of these children had a developmental language disorder and associated focal IEDs without a direct causal link. In some similar cases followed without any therapy, the IEDs persist while language gradually improves, suggesting that they were independent elements of an underlying disorder of cerebral maturation. However limited, these data confirm that early age of onset is only one of the several variables that will influence the long-term outcome of LKS. They also mean that early and prolonged language delay and impairment during several years does not preclude a fair outcome.

8
FROM ROLANDIC EPILEPSY TO LANDAU–KLEFFNER SYNDROME

Introduction

The study of the continuum between rolandic epilepsy and Landau–Kleffner syndrome (LKS) is our starting point for thinking about acquired language and other disturbances that can be found in these epilepsies. As discussed in the historical section (Chapter 2), it took some time to recognize that children with rolandic epilepsy could have from onset or later on epileptic foci in another than the centrotemporal location, that these foci could be bilateral or multiple, that they could propagate locally or more diffusely and get variably activated during sleep. At the same time, the importance of the role of both hemispheres in speech and language development was gradually uncovered.

Rolandic seizures are the most 'visible' among the focal epileptic manifestations that arise within the 'perisylvian' region. These consist of hemifacial and oropharyngeal sensory-motor manifestations that mainly occur in transitional states between wakefulness and sleep. They are often followed by a brief post-ictal period of anarthria or speech production deficit. Their electroencephalogram (EEG) correlate is an age-limited paroxysmal bioelectric instability of the perisylvian region centred on the lower rolandic area, the so-called centrotemporal spikes or focal sharp wave (FSW) (see Chapter 9).

If the focal seizure activity is located in a more posterior temporal region such as the auditory cortices, there may be no 'positive' clinical manifestation: The child may experience a temporary deficit in auditory-language processing that can be recognized only when listening to sounds, speech, speaking or reading. Positive phenomena such as auditory hallucinations may also occur (see below and Chapter 5). The function of the cortex where the main epileptic focus arises will thus determine the nature of the clinical symptoms, whereas its intensity, local, bilateral or more distant spread via pre-established pathways will contribute to the overall picture.

The perisylvian regions are genetically programmed to support all structural components of human verbal communication in collaboration with adjacent cortical areas (parietal and frontal) and subcortical structures. The complexity of the language network (see Chapter 4, Hickok & Poeppel model) may reflect its key importance in human language, a late appearing function in phylogeny, meaning more than understanding and signalling short immediate messages but the exchange knowledge, ideas and feelings.

The elaborate and scheduled organization of this unique human function may explain a focal imbalance between excitatory and inhibitory processes in these perisylvian regions during the childhood years of language network patterning and stabilization, resulting in a propensity to generate local and age-limited epileptic phenomena (Halasz et al. 2005). Genes involved in this refined organization may be mutated resulting in alteration of the function assumed by the network – here speech and language – and/or its excitatory threshold.

Typical rolandic epilepsy: evolution, cognition, behaviour and learning

A first step is to review the clinical data on the neuropsychological, electrophysiological, genetic and more recently functional imaging studies data that have accumulated in recent years in rolandic epilepsies.

COGNITIVE DEVELOPMENT AND LONG-TERM OUTCOME

The vast majority of children with rolandic epilepsy will ultimately have a normal cognitive outcome, meaning that, as adults, they will statistically not have more difficulties than the normal population (Loiseau 1983; Hommet 2001). Such comparisons were based on gross indices such as employment or certification in regular schools. Prolonged academic or behavioural difficulties during childhood, even if subsequently overcome may be of significance and leave permanent emotional and other traces. This is emphasized here, because some epileptologists tend to minimize this dimension and think that reassurance of the final overall good prognosis of the epilepsy is all that counts.

Over the years, it has become gradually clear that learning or behavioural impairments are a frequent component of the rolandic epilepsy phenotype (see below and Vannest et al. 2015, for a recent and exhaustive review). Previously, the behavioural and/or school impairments were easily misunderstood as being primarily psychological, given the child's normal intelligence and good capacities in many domains (Beaussart 1972). Several studies have later shown that children with rolandic epilepsy often have a mild oromotor–speech immaturity, speech–sound and auditory processing impairments compared to typically developing children (Lundberg et al. 2005). More recently, difficulties with written language learning and behavioural problems have been recognized, while subtle deficits in executive functions and social cognition are now also being suspected (Deltour et al. 2007; Sarco et al. 2011; Neri et al. 2012; Kwon 2012; Genizi 2012; Filippini 2016). Siblings of children with rolandic epilepsy who never had seizures have been found in some studies to have the same or even worse scores in some neuropsychological tests. This has given some weight to the concept that a genetic developmental abnormality or 'immaturity' is at the basis of these disorders, and not, or not only, the epilepsy per se (the 'hereditary impairment of brain maturation' of Doose 1996; Pal 2011; Smith et al. 2012; Verrotti et al. 2013).

However, most of the controlled studies on cognition and behaviour in children with rolandic epilepsy were done at the time of diagnosis or, more often, months or years later and were cross sectional. The children were of varying ages at seizure onset often with EEGs performed long before the neuropsychological tests. In addition, participants did or did not take antiepileptic medications at the time of study. In these conditions, interpretation is problematic at two levels. The first is neuropsychological: It is difficult to ascertain that variations in language-related skills such as reading and writing that are often minor in comparison with controls are specifically of linguistic nature. They may be due to other cognitive or behavioural variables such as inattention or impulsivity. The second is aetiological: The design of these studies can neither affirm nor deny a direct role of the epileptic activity in the observed deficits. These studies were however an important first step in the recognition of previously neglected difficulties, whatever be their cause (Staden et al. 1998; Northcott et al. 2005; Clarke et al. 2007; Danielsson and Petermann 2009; Jurkeviciene et al. 2012; Verrotti et al. 2013).

When a child is first diagnosed with rolandic epilepsy, he/she may actually already have unrecognized seizures or focal IEDs for some time that may have influenced development behaviour and cognition as shown in Figure 8.1.

Most children continue to develop within the normal range that is sketched in the 'corridor.' (dotted lines in the figure), representing normal cognitive development (see Fig 8.1 upper part). In a minority, epilepsy could have influenced the optimal development of some specific language -related or other skills: This may explain a temporary cognitive decline before or after the time of diagnosis (curved arrows within and below the 'corridor'). A mild slowing or regression can sometimes occur (curved arrow) in the active phase of the epilepsy (seizures and EEG findings), but is often only recognized in retrospect, when the child's epilepsy abates. Baseline development can be in the upper or lower normal range, either causally related to the epilepsy or not.

The finding of a positive correlation between the location (centrotemporal vs. more posterior) of the main epileptic focus found by magnetoencephalography and the nature of the cognitive dysfunction (verbal vs. visuospatial) in cases of otherwise typical rolandic

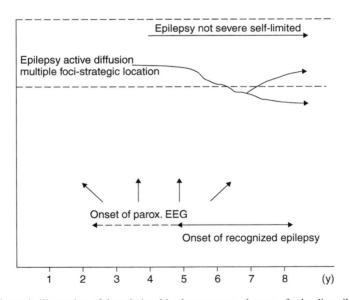

Fig. 8.1. Schematic illustration of the relationships between actual onset of rolandic epilepsy clinical diagnosis and the possible consequences on cognitive functions (see explanation in text). From Deonna T and Roulet-Perez E, Cognitive and Behavioural Disorders of Epileptic Origin in Children, CDM No. 168. London: Mac Keith Press, 2005, p 96.

epilepsy is an indication that both are tightly connected (Wolff et al. 2005). This however does not prove a direct contribution of the epilepsy, unless changes are shown to be reversible with time and correlated with EEG findings (Metz-Lutz et al. 1999).

In a follow-up study of a cohort of 26 children with rolandic epilepsy, Lindgren et al. (2004) re-assessed the same patients tested by Croona et al. (1999) 2 years and 6 months to 3 years before with the same neuropsychological test battery: they found that most of the previously pathological results normalized except verbal fluency and word reading comprehension. General IQ and non-verbal reasoning was the same as in controls, as well as the ability for immediate memory, learning of auditory-verbal and visuospatial material and delayed recall. The everyday functioning at home and at school was not affected. EEG was unfortunately not performed at the time of assessment, and half of the patients were still on medication, so that the real contribution of the epileptic activity versus maturational, compensatory or other factors cannot be disentangled.

A few prospective studies provide details of the children's cognitive performances at onset, during the active epilepsy course and after EEG normalization or improvement and suggest a possible direct negative influence of the paroxysmal EEG discharges (Deonna 2001; Baglietto et al. 2001). In our own longitudinal study (Deonna 2001) of 22 children, eight children had transient weak scores in one isolated cognitive function (verbal, visuospatial, memory) that improved or normalized during the course of the study with concomittant EEG improvement or normalization. Baglietto et al. (2001) made a 2-year follow-up correlative neuropsychological–EEG study (with controls) of nine children with rolandic epilepsy with marked activation of IEDs during sleep. At the time of IED remission, reevaluation showed a notable increase in IQ scores and a significant improvement in visuomotor coordination, non-verbal short-term memory, sustained attention and mental flexibility, picture naming and visual-perceptual performance. In a recent extensive review on cognitive and behavioural outcomes in children with rolandic epilepsy (Vannest et al. 2015), the authors state: 'Longitudinal data from patients with rolandic epilepsy including serial EEG, neuroimaging and cognitive testing would help clarify the interaction among these factors, e.g., whether improvements in cognitive/behavioral outcomes are associated with reduction of centrotemporal spikes.' This seems evident, but is still rarely followed advice. Ewen et al. (2011) made a prospective study of six children with rolandic epilepsy tested 3 times at 4-5 week interval. It showed significant cognitive and EEG fluctuations. However, the study had several methodological shortcomings well acknowledged by the authors. It did not allow a definite conclusion on the direct role of epileptic activity (Ewen 2011), but is a good step in that direction.

Brain anatomy and organization in children with rolandic epilepsy
All the above-mentioned studies have to be interpreted in the context of a child's individual epilepsy history (seizure and/or EEG) before the first evaluation, a variable that can influence brain development and organization.

Although clinical MRI studies of patients with rolandic epilepsy show no lesion, advanced neuroimaging has started to bring out subtle variations in brain morphology in several cortical regions (Pardoe et al. 2013). The authors concluded that there was an age-dependant alteration of the trajectory of normal development in some regions of the cortex, mainly in frontal and to a lesser extent in parietal and insular regions. They argued that these regions extend beyond the centro-temporal areas that are generating the spikes, so that increased regional volume was unlikely to be the consequence of the epileptic activity. This study has of course its methodological limits (technical issues, cross-sectional and not longitudinal design, absence of data on epilepsy variables, propagation patterns, absence of language and other neuropsychological data). However, it is an example of the increasing contribution of technological advances in brain morphology imaging to our understanding of rolandic epilepsy and epilepsy aphasia spectrum.

Regarding functional organization of language, already in 1988, the findings of Piccirilli et al. of atypical language lateralization in children with rolandic epilepsy and a left-sided focus using a neuropsychological approach (dual-task) suggested a modified hemispheric organization in this population. This issue has continued to be studied with newer methods (dichotic listening: Bulgheroni et al. 2008; Lillywhite; functional MRI, Lillywhite et al. 2009; Event-related potentials Monjauze et al. 2011; functional MRI, Datta et al. 2013a) and confirmed that language organization (or reorganization) actually takes place in bilateral or right hemispheric language networks. For instance, Datta et al. (2013a) studied 27 children with rolandic epilepsy via language functional MRI using a silent simple sentence generation and a silent word-pair paradigm and found more bilateral hemispheric activation than in controls, especially in the anterior part of the language network.

Again, whether the findings from these different studies reflect a developmental brain variation or anomaly of the language networks or results from persistent focal or multifocal interictal discharges that gradually modify the initial 'standard' organization plan remains open to question. Most studies have not been performed at disease onset (Bulgheroni: 9y 5mo; Lillywhite: 9y 2mo; Monjauze: 18y). Only when a change in language organization in correlation with the localization of the epileptic activity can be demonstrated prospectively can one conclude that this has been acquired because of the epileptic activity. The first case suggesting that such a change can indeed happen was reported in a single case study by Datta et al. (2013a). In a child with a typical left-sided rolandic epilepsy that evolved into LKS (see p. 89) a functional MRI showed a change in language dominance from left to right hemisphere within the year following acquired verbal auditory agnosia.

Using tractography, Besseling et al. (2013) showed reduced structural connectivity between sensorimotor and language areas in a cohort of 23 children with rolandic epilepsy compared to controls. This finding correlated with overall language competences. Besides innate structural abnormalities or epilepsy-induced underdevelopment, this could also be the consequence of language under use.

Taken together, all these data suggest that the brain of children with rolandic epilepsy may have an innate functional brain organization in the perisylvian region that is different from controls. It generates a focal/multifocal epileptic activity that can still further modify this organization and result in suboptimal or abnormal language function, especially when early, bilateral and sustained. However, some children with rolandic epilepsy could have a 'standard' developmental brain organization to begin with, but that can undergo changes due to the epileptic activity. Both possibilities are not mutually exclusive. Given this atypical language organization and the recurrent and switching focal epileptic activity from a location to another at different developmental periods, one must expect that the cognitive consequences are more variable than in children with a fixed focal epileptogenic lesion.

Rolandic epilepsy and LKS: the continuum within the perisylvian region

It is not unusual, but rarely mentioned or underlined, that children diagnosed with LKS can have a history of rolandic epilepsy or of not further precised 'nocturnal seizures', sometimes just a single one. This can occur long before language regression sets in but also during its course, or even after the aphasia had resolved.

We observed this in the child (GA) described in Chapter 5 with a relatively brief period of aphasia who, after recovery, described and drew the hemifacial seizures he had on awakening. These occurred only in the early morning and persisted for 3 years without relapse of the language deficit.

One can thus suspect that children with LKS whose family never reported seizures may still have had unrecognized clinical manifestations related to the centrotemporal region.

More recently, systematic follow-up studies of children presenting initially with classic rolandic epilepsy (Fejerman et al. 2000; Tovia et al. 2011) an estimated of 5%–10% of these cases had a complicated course with acquired cognitive–behavioural deficits including LKS. One must stress that only children with significant acquired language and/or other cognitive disturbances would be included in such studies.

A table summarizing shared feature between LKS and rolandic epilepsy can be found in the Chapter 2, Table 2.3.

Rolandic epilepsy with acquired oromotor and speech deficits: 'acquired epileptic opercular syndrome'
Some children with initially typical rolandic epilepsy can develop dysfunction of the bucco-linguo-facial and pharyngeal movements that may result, when severe, in inability to swallow and speak. Unlike the short post-ictal deficit often reported by parents after a rolandic seizure,

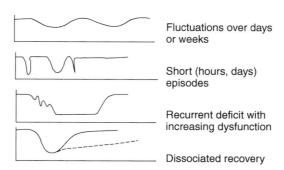

Fluctuations over days or weeks

Short (hours, days) episodes

Recurrent deficit with increasing dysfunction

Dissociated recovery

Fig. 8.2. Rolandic epilepsy with acquired oromotor ('acquired epileptic opercular syndrome') and speech deficits. (From Deonna T and Roulet-Perez T. Cognitive and Behavioural Disorders of Epiliptic Origin in Children. Clinics in Deveopmental Medicine No. 167. London: Mac Keith Press, 2005. p 89.)

this deficit can last for hours, days and weeks. On the EEG, it is associated with increased daytime epileptic activity in both lower rolandic areas that merges into CSWS during the night. These are striking examples of an acquired sustained 'neurological' (as opposed to cognitive) manifestation of epilepsy. The dynamics of installation, duration, progression and recovery of these oromotor and speech disturbances in children with rolandic epilepsy was closely observed in three personal cases and six from the literature (see case reports, Roulet et al. 1989; Deonna 1993; de Saint-Martin et al. 1999). Severity and time course of the manifestations in these patients differed and are schematized in Figure 8.2 (Deonna 1993).

These children can present with drooling, difficulties with chewing and sometimes with swallowing, so that they have to be tube-fed (Boulloche et al. 1990; case 2, Lou et al. 1977). Drooling and lingual dyspraxia can be seen without speech difficulties (Roulet et al. 1989). Decreased facial mobility and unawareness of the presence of food in the mouth can be additional features (Roulet et al. 1989). The latter is referred to as 'oral sensory agnosia' (Shafrir and Prensky 1995). It may appear surprising that it took so long to report such cases and to realize that the mode of onset, fluctuating clinical course, sleep-activated EEG abnormalities, including CSWS and response to steroids, were actually very similar to LKS (Deonna 1993). As with LKS, some of these children did not have seizures before their neurological deficit did set in. One case even seemed to have a normal awake and sleep EEG during a relapse (Arslan et al. 2012), adding to the diagnostic difficulty, but information on the type of record (whole night versus nap EEG) was not provided. Interestingly, oromotor involvement was already reported during the fluctuating course of LKS with VAA (Lou et al. 1977) in a patient who went through a phase of drooling and inability to feed himself late in the course of the disorder.

In these cases, labelled 'acquired epileptiform opercular syndrome' (Colamaria et al. 1991; Shafrir and Prensky 1995), that we will designate here 'acquired epileptic opercular syndrome' (AEOS) by analogy with 'acquired epileptic aphasia', the loss of intelligible speech is attributed to dysarthria secondary to the oromotor impairment. An additional phonological programming deficit or an aphasic component (anomia) may sometimes also contribute to the clinical picture, but can only be recognized when the dysarthria subsides. It probably varies with the extent of the epileptic dysfunction in anatomically closely related perisylvian networks (Deonna 1993).

In 1999, de Saint-Martin et al. published a prospective longitudinal study of a girl who started with rolandic seizures at the age of 3 years 6 months and presented three periods of several weeks of clinical worsening between ages 5 and 6: each of these periods was characterized by an increased frequency of diurnal rolandic seizures followed by a short lived unilateral facial paresis, brief facial myoclonic jerks and a prolonged but fluctuating oromotor deficit (drooling, bilateral facial weakness, dysarthria and dysphagia). Behavioural changes were also noted. The EEG showed bilateral independent centrotemporal foci with major activation during sleep (corresponding to CSWS during the two first periods, but not the last). A brain MRI was normal. The child was first treated with valproic acid, substituted by clobazam after the second period of worsening. After a last adjustment of the dose to 1.5mg/kg/day, her epilepsy remitted with disappearance of the EEG abnormalities until the end of follow-up at the age of 7 years 9 months. The child recovered full oromotor function.

A first neuropsychological assessment at the age of 4 years 10 months, that is, after seizure onset but before the first phase of worsening, showed altered articulation of speech, poor lexical abilities, and impaired short-term auditory memory. Her full-scale IQ (Wechsler Preschool and Primary Scale of Intelligence) was 78 (verbal IQ, 86; performance IQ, 74). After remission, when neurological examination and oromotor function had normalized (after the age of 6, precise age not given), her full scale IQ was 82 (verbal IQ, 79; performance IQ, 85) and her verbal short-term memory performances had almost normalized.

This illustrates the point that during the prodromal phase of AEOS there was already a deficit that did not purely affect speech production but also higher level language functions. This was presumably acquired because the child had a normal developmental history, and no regression in speech was mentioned. During the active phase of the disease, the authors were actually able to demonstrate hypermetabolism in the frontal opercular areas in addition to both rolandic cortices via a Fludeoxyglucose-postitron emission tomography (FDG-PET) study. These findings and the detailed EEG studies are discussed in Chapter 10.

Many similar cases have been published since the 1990s, sometimes without firm opinion on their nosological place (Shuper 2000; Tachikawa et al. 2001; Kubota et al. 2004; Tohyama et al. 2011; Arslan et al. 2012) and thus giving the impression of a separate entity instead of belonging to a continuum with rolandic epilepsy, LKS and ECSWS. They can also be found in follow-up studies of rolandic epilepsy (Fejerman et al. 2000; Kramer et al. 2001; Saltik et al. 2005; Tovia et al. 2011) or of children with ECSWS (Veggiotti et al. 1999). Analysis of the clinical symptoms and of the rare clinical-EEG correlations and functional imaging data in all these publications allow us to see a combination of the various dynamics of installation and duration the epilepsy-related deficits, as illustrated in Figure 8.2 (see also Chapter 10).

Tohyama et al. (2011) reported a girl with a severe fluctuating oromotor dysfunction and dysarthria from the age of 7 to 10 years – two years after a single convulsion – and a diagnosis of rolandic epilepsy. MEG analysis showed broadly distributed epileptic foci around the sylvian fissure, including a secondary contralateral source. About their first MEG study at the age of 7 years and 7 months, the authors note that 'current dipoles of the left hemisphere were localized in the prerolandic area, presumably indicating the premotor cortex. Current dipoles of the right hemisphere were localized around the central sulcus and sylvian fissure'. A follow-up MEG study 1 year later showed a change in location of the dipole which was found more posteriorly, illustrating the propensity of these epileptic foci to migrate or appear in other locations. At the age of 16, this patient demonstrated 'no dysarthria or oromotor deficit and prednisolone was stopped', indicating that despite their long duration and severity, these oromotor and motor speech deficits can be clinically reversible.

ROLANDIC EPILEPSY WITH ACQUIRED EPILEPTIC DYSGRAPHIA

Besides oral language, an acquired deficit of writing, a later learned fine motor and linguistic skill, is an example of the variety and selectivity of higher cortical functions that can be temporarily involved at different ages (Halasz et al. 2005), and easily escape recognition.

In 1993, we published a longitudinal case study (Mayor-Dubois et al. 2003; Deonna and Roulet-Perez 2005, pp. 91–92) of a boy who presented at 7 years with a typical rolandic epilepsy: He developed a selective handwriting impairment which was serially documented via a computerized writing pad. At the age of 11, several parameters of the graphomotor act like velocity and precision were analyzed and compared with controls at the age of 11. The child's handwriting disorder was neither explained by focal negative myoclonus, writer's cramp, nor a sensorimotor deficit of the right hand. Neither was there impulsivity or a visuospatial deficit. The writing deficit was not associated with focal motor seizures, but correlated with the worsening of the EEG. The records showed bilateral focal sharp waves with variable increase of frequency and diffusion during sleep but not CSWS in the strict sense. The child had no orthographic difficulties, except for brief period of sound–letter conversion errors that correlated with a worsening of the epileptic activity on the EEG and subsided with its normalization. The child's graphomotor skills had been considered normal until the epilepsy started, then slowed down and regressed rapidly at the age of 11. Significant improvement was rapid but only partial within a few weeks coincident with spontaneous reduction of EEG discharges and subsequently continued over the next two years to almost normal.

In an unpublished study by Rejnö-Habte Selassie and Uvebrant, a child who presented with a prolonged but reversible severe speech deficit amounting to mutism, a simultaneous loss of graphomotor skills was also observed and evolved in parallel (see Chapter 14).

Both cases illustrate how rolandic epilepsy can interfere either selectively or simultaneous with functionally and anatomically closely related networks supporting graphomotor, oromotor and speech programming skills.

IDIOPATHIC FOCAL EPILEPSY WITH INTERMITTENT INCREASE IN READING DIFFICULTIES

'Laurent' was first seen by us at the age of 6 years and 6 months after a first nocturnal seizure. His development was normal, but he had been evaluated by a child psychiatrist because of behavioural problems. An EEG showed a left temporal electrical seizure and independent bilateral frontotemporal focal sharp waves. A brain MRI was normal. A diagnosis of idiopathic focal epilepsy, possibly a variant of rolandic epilepsy was made. In the following months, the mother and teacher noted periods of agitation, intermittent worsening of reading skills and occasional nocturnal urinary incontinence. Neuropsychological testing at 7 years and 6 months showed normal oral language and cognitive abilities but a specific delay in reading acquisition. At 8 years, comparative videotapes of the child while reading aloud the same text, obtained two weeks apart (one recorded at school by the teacher during the reported 'bad' phase, and the other by the mother at home in a baseline period) were analysed. During the 'bad period' there were (1) fluctuations of performances across the session, (2) slow reading speed, (3) inaccuracies with many mistakes in word reading, (4) words far from target and (5) omission of grammatical words. All these difficulties were not present two weeks later when he was considered back to 'normal' by family and teacher. Importantly, there was no simultaneous difficulty with oral language and behaviour, so that this would have passed unnoticed if reading aloud had not been practised regularly at school and at home. Behavioural problems, urinary incontinence and fluctuations in reading disappeared and the EEG normalized after introduction of sulthiame (STM). He never had seizure relapses and no reading problems at the last follow-up at 13. He attended mainstream school with specific help in written language (mainly spelling). Although this child probably already had some difficulties in learning to read before the epilepsy started, there was a definite transient epilepsy-related worsening of this capacity. The single nocturnal seizure, the focal sharp waves on the EEG, the rapid clinical and EEG response to sulthiame therapy and complete long-term remission are in keeping with an idiopathic focal epilepsy within the EAS spectrum.

Rolandic epilepsy with acquired language deficits: from mild acquired language disturbances to fully-developed LKS

Another instance of the continuity between rolandic epilepsy and LKS is the child who starts with typical rolandic seizures and later develops language comprehension difficulties (VAA). Actually, the same child may first present with an acquired oromotor impairment and subsequently with language comprehension difficulties, depending on shifts in the localization and/or propagation pattern of the focal epileptic activity. We know of several cases of this kind of evolution; however, this is rarely documented precisely.

TYPICAL ROLANDIC EPILEPSY EVOLVING TO LKS DOCUMENTED VIA EEG AND FUNCTIONAL IMAGING: A LONG-AWAITED DECISIVE PROSPECTIVE STUDY

Datta et al.'s (2013b) study is to our knowledge the first demonstrating that the evolution from rolandic epilepsy to LKS correlated with a shift in the predominant location of the focal interictal EEG activity with bilateral involvement and sleep activation of IEDs. This

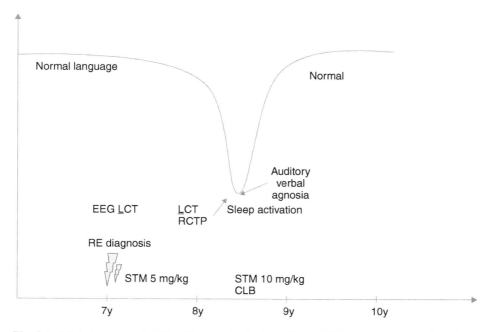

Fig. 8.3. Clinical course of child with typical rolandic epilepsy (RE) evolving to verbal auditory agnosia. LCT, left centrotemporal; RCTP: right centrotemporoparietal; STM: sulthiame; CLB: clobazam. Adapted from Datta et al. 2013b.

is illustrated in Figure 8.3 drawn from the data and EEG illustrations provided in the paper. It was fortunate that Datta et al. had the opportunity to study this unique case with EEG, source imaging that allows more precise localization of the epileptic foci. Hence, he was able to demonstrate what was suspected for a long time. It is nevertheless surprising that it took so long to have the first clear prospective clinical- EEG demonstration of this evolution (see Chapter 2).

ROLANDIC EPILEPSY EVOLVING INTO MILD LKS: AN EASILY MISSED SITUATION

A situation in which a moderate LKS could escape recognition is when a child with rolandic epilepsy and a history of developmental speech delay becomes behaviourally disturbed, hyperactive and oppositional. Many other explanations than a worsening of his epilepsy can be put forward if language is not assessed. The following case report (Korff, Deonna, unpublished) is an eloquent example.

At the age of 4, this boy had four episodes of hemifacial seizures within a month. His EEG showed bilateral centrotemporal discharges with left-sided predominance. He was put on valproic acid (VPA) and did not have other seizures. At the age of 6, the family moved from Portugal to Geneva where he rapidly learned French. At the age of 7, he again had a few seizures and presented a behavioural and language deterioration noted in Portuguese and French. At the age of 7 years and 6 months, a repeat EEG showed frequent FSW in the left centrotemporal region with occasional diffusion to the right and activation during slow wave sleep (30%–40% of the tracing). At this time, he had no medication. Neuropsychological examination showed poor comprehension with major word repetition difficulties (0 out of 12 words) and reduced, sometimes almost unintelligible productions. He also had a major attention deficit and sleep difficulties and he failed at school. Clobazam (5mg) at night was started and his sleep and behaviour improved within 10 days, followed by recovery of language comprehension and almost fluent speech. A whole night control EEG 3 months after the introduction of clobazam showed the disappearance of the epileptiform discharges. One month later, he was able to understand a simple conversation, could repeat 3–4 syllables words. Repeat questioning of the mother disclosed that he actually had a 2-year period of fluctuating speech disturbances after seizure onset at 4 years. These were in retrospect quite similar, but less severe than when the seizure relapsed at the age of 7 years.

A difficult family situation, associated attentional–behavioural problems and the recently learned foreign language explained that the initial fluctuating milder deficits were not recognized.

SHORT-LIVED CENTRAL AUDITORY DISTURBANCES IN THE COURSE OF ROLANDIC EPILEPSY: LKS, 'A MINIMA'

As discussed at the beginning of this chapter, children in whom the epileptic activity involves the auditory cortex and remains self-limited in time and location may only present auditory hallucinations or temporary auditory processing deficits.

An exceptional example of this situation was studied in detail and presented at several meetings but unfortunately never published (Metz-Lutz 2009). It is presented here with permission.

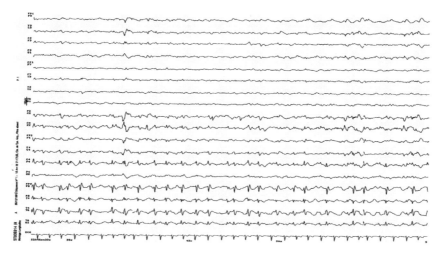

Fig. 8.4. Waking EEG showing right temporal spikes. (EEG courtesy of Marie-Noëlle Metz-Lutz.)

A 6-year-6-month-old right-handed girl was referred for a single nocturnal generalized seizure. In the previous weeks, she had three short episodes of hearing loss with right ear buzzing and, on one occasion, naming difficulties. The waking EEG recorded showed paroxysmal spike wave discharges centred on T4 (Fig 8.4).

The neuropsychological examination did not disclose any verbal expressive or receptive impairment. She had a full IQ of 122. Auditory event-related potentials recorded showed normal amplitude and latencies of the early components at all stimulus intensities. The mid-latency component of the left ear however showed abnormal responses peaking at 20 ms. Vocal and tonal audiograms were normal for both ears. A dichotic listening task revealed right-left discrepancy in reporting pairs of digits presented simultaneously to both ears. She had no difficulty in identifying non-speech sounds. Phonological discrimination tasks remained unimpaired as well as verbal short term and working memory.

FDG-PET performed during the same active period of epiletiform discharges disclosed a focal increase of FDG uptake restricted to the right superior temporal gyrus in BA 22.

It is difficult to know exactly what type of central auditory deficit this child had, because she had already clinically recovered by the time of testing. The nocturnal seizure, typical EEG abnormalities and good long-term follow-up is otherwise fully in keeping with the diagnosis of rolandic epilepsy. The hypermetabolic focus on the PET in the right temporal region was likely to be due to the intense focal IEDs (Chapter 11, De Tiège).

The authors of this remarkable study were able to demonstrate, despite the very short course and essentially subjective complaints what we can consider a 'minima' form of LKS that resolved spontaneously. The 'buzzing' in the ear was probably a simple auditory hallucination as was reported in a child of our (see, child GA in Chapter 5) and by

Morrell et al. (1995) in his prolonged video-recorded clinical and EEG studies at different periods of their LKS.

We have occasionally heard from our colleagues about a child with rolandic epilepsy who had a phase of transient speech-language impairment that never relapsed and for which different explanations had been put forward. In our longitudinal follow-up study of 22 children with rolandic epilepsy, one child had such a history. Another child had transient written language difficulties that correlated with a worsening of the epileptic activity on the EEG (Deonna 2001). Similar transient deficits were also found in a recent longitudinal EEG (including sleep records) and neuropsychological study of 33 children with rolandic epilepsy (Filippini et al. 2013). Two participants who were initially tested as normal subsequently presented a transient language deficit affecting 'phonological decoding and lexical retrieval'. The authors labelled these cases 'mild transitory language difficulties without a real regression'. Unfortunately, no EEG was obtained during these periods, and it is difficult to state that these transient deficits were epilepsy-related or not. We would also consider these cases as possible 'a minima' LKS and include them in the EAS spectrum. Typically, developing children will never present with an acquired but reversible phonological decoding or word finding difficulties, unless there is a precise reason. Besides an epileptic dysfunction, explanations could be hypoacousis due to middle ear effusion or a word-finding difficulty related to an antiepileptic or another drug (Battaglia et al. 2001). An alternative explanation could be that a child with a just compensated previous developmental language disorder becomes again symptomatic with fatigue or stress related to the epilepsy or a non-specific effect of an anti-epileptic drug (AED). There is no definite answer for Filipiini 's two cases (personal communication with the authors, 2015), but this situation illustrates how difficult it is to demonstrate the existence of minor and transient epilepsy-related language impairment within the AES spectrum, unless correlating clinical/language and EEG data are obtained prospectively.

Autosomal dominant rolandic epilepsy and speech dyspraxia

Twenty years ago, an original and influential paper by Scheffer et al. (1995) reported the co-occurrence of rolandic epilepsy and speech dyspraxia running as a dominant trait in a large Australian family. The authors proposed the view that the speech disorder and the epilepsy were separate features of the inherited disease autosomal dominant rolandic epilepsy and speech dyspraxia (ADRESD), a new syndrome (1995).

Recently a mutation in *GRIN2A* was found in this family and other families with a similar clinical phenotype within the AES (see Chapter 9).

The relative contribution of an innate speech and language versus an early acquired epilepsy-related disturbance component may be further examined with Scheffer's and the other rare reported families with the ADRESD phenotype. The proband of Scheffer's family probably suffered from nocturnal rolandic seizures since the age of 2 years and 6 months and was first seen by the authors at the age of 5 with what one would now call AEOS: he had fluctuating drooling, stuttering, unintelligible speech and oromotor and general motor disturbances. The corresponding EEG records showed continuous bilateral predominantly right-sided centrotemporal discharges during the waking and sleep state, but not the ictal tracing of rolandic seizures. The brain MRI was normal, including the opercular regions, which were scrutinized for a possible polymicrogyria or dysplasia. Only one assessment of oromotor, speech and other cognitive functions was provided, and it is unclear when it was performed in relation to the continuous epileptic activity (recurrence at 6 and 7 years). The authors report a previous developmental delay but do not describe the child's motor, speech and language development except that 'he spoke only a single word at 21 months'. Speech improved after valproate was introduced without further details. All other affected family members had rolandic seizures with a typical EEG when available. The father of the proband had a speech delay before the onset of seizure, whereas the father's twin brother, who also had rolandic epilepsy, had normal development. One family member had a speech dyspraxia without a history of seizures, but he was from the older generation (proband's grandfather) and there was no reliable information on his childhood.

In our opinion, albeit the proband and some of his relatives appear to have a pre-existing developmental speech disorder, it is likely that part of the neuropsychological phenotype (including low IQ) was acquired and related to the early onset of active and prolonged bilateral rolandic IEDs.

Since Scheffer's publication, there has been only two large multiplex families reported with a closely resembling constellation (Roll et al. 2006; Kugler et al. 2008). In the family reported by Roll, a *GRIN2A* mutation was ultimately found and the role of the initially reported *SRPX2* mutation can be questioned (Lesca et al. 2013; Turner et al. 2015a, b). In Kugler's family, the proband was a 7-year-old boy with rolandic seizures from the age of 6. There was 'no history of oromotor problems in infancy', but 'since early childhood he had severe difficulties in speech production and fine motor control'. His father (34y) had onset of rolandic seizures at 3 years and 'he reported marked difficulties with speech in childhood' and 'had learning difficulties at school'. The proband's second cousin was a 12 years old with 'speech and language delay and slow speech with no sentences until 3 to 4 years of age'. His first seizures started at 2 years and 6 months. These are the best available pieces of information on early speech and language development. At follow-up, it is stated: 'In acoustic analysis of three adult members, there was only marginal evidence of residual speech dyspraxia'. In comparison 'two subjects showed evidence of severe oromotor apraxia' (presumably the proband and his 12-year-old second cousin). Differences from Scheffer's family were 'minimal residual evidence of speech dyspraxia' (Kugler et al. 2008), a longer course of the epilepsy and lack of aggravation from the first generation to the next suggesting genetic anticipation. Like Scheffer's, Kugler et al.'s (2008) conclusion was about segregation of the phenotype. Patient 'III-5 has a mild seizure phenotype and while one of her parent had both epilepsy and speech impairment, another has only inherited speech impairment, suggesting that the two symptoms are independent'.

Another publication that takes an opposite stance and argues in favour of a role of the epilepsy in the severity of the phenotype was published by Prats et al. (1999) entitled as 'Opercular epileptic syndrome: an unusual form of benign epilepsy in childhood'. The study went unnoticed probably because it was written in Spanish and did not mention the familial aspect in its title. The authors reported four patients, three of whom being a father and his two children. In all cases, oromotor and speech disturbances started with typical rolandic seizures and continued with fluctuations for a prolonged period. They were described as 'severe drooling, facial hypomobility, and speech disturbances which waxed and vanished in weeks, months or years, apparently not post-ictal'. One patient was aggravated by carbamazepine. There was no history of developmental oromotor and speech difficulties. The father had benign neonatal convulsions (like his sister) and at 3 years 3 months, he developed difficulties in moving his tongue and in pronouncing words. These oromotor deficits fluctuated but persisted for several years. Difficulties in moving his tongue and perioral musculature were still present after adolescence, long after remission of the epilepsy. He attended mainstream school and graduated from university. Prats's cases suggest that early onset severe prolonged rolandic epilepsy can leave permanent sequelae, and that these are not primarily related to an associated developmental speech disorder.

In summary, all these data suggest that in the context of rolandic epilepsy the epileptic activity in the lower rolandic cortex can lead to arrest, stagnation or regression of functions related to the anterior opercular region, that is, oromotor functions and/or speech execution and programming skills. When earlier than usually seen in rolandic epilepsy, this dysfunction may mimic a developmental 'speech delay' and normalize or lead to permanent oromotor and speech dyspraxia (see Chapter 6, Julian). To what extent the acquired deficit is superimposed on genetically determined a pre-existing delayed or abnormal development of these functions remains an open question.

Prospective studies of further ADRESD families scrutinizing early development and EEG findings as well as looking for dissociated speech – epilepsy phenotypes in patients harbouring a known genetic mutation – may help to clarify this issue. This may be facilitated now that large-scale genetic studies are increasingly performed in cohorts with rolandic epilepsy and EASs and in cohorts with speech and language disorders (see Chapter 9).

Acquired epileptic frontal syndrome in the context of rolandic epilepsy and EAS syndromes: beyond the perisylvian region

Rare children initially having a typical rolandic epilepsy or another IFE may later present with a severe cognitive and behavioral regression with failure to learn. At this time, CSWS are often found and epileptic foci are merely located in the frontal or fronto-temporal rather than the centro-temporal regions, at times multiple and shifting.

In these cases, speech and language can be preserved or at least not affected predominantly: altered production and comprehension can result from severe executive deficits with lack of initiative or monitoring of language output and thought process (Kyllerman 1996). Patients may for instance be mute (or nearly so) or produce neologisms and sentences with a disorganized syntax and content. When these improve, language appears preserved in its formal aspects, albeit its content, pragmatics and verbal reasoning can remain poor (Roulet–Perez 1993).

Severe attention deficit, hyperactivity, impulsivenss, disinhibition, perseverative behaviors and mood changes are core clinical features. We coined the term 'acquired epileptic frontal syndrome' for these cases, referring mainly to this striking clinical picture. The course can be long lasting with behavioral and neuropsychological improvement after the active period of the epilepsy (CSWS), but patients often harbor permanent sequelae in adulthood ranging from intellectual disability to borderline-normal IQ (Veggiotti 2001; Praline et al. 2003; Pera et al. 2013). In our own adult follow-up study, executive and behavioral difficulties were no more in the forefront (Seegmüller 2012).

This pattern of 'acquired epileptic frontal syndrome' can be of variable severity and actually occur in the active (CSWS) phase of any epilepsy within the EAS. It may add to or mask other deficits, like specific language deficits (see Chapter 5, p.56). It is also a feature of frontal epilepsy of unknown origin (Matricardi et al. 2016) and in lesional ECSWS (Kallay et al. 2009). In IFE and the EAS syndromes, acquired executive cognitive and behavioral disturbances may either result from a focal epileptic dysfunction – for instance shifting of a centro-temporal focus to the prefrontal regions or apparition of new, independent foci in these regions- or result from propagation of the perisylvian epileptic activity towards the prefrontal regions via more remotely connected neural newtworks (See Chapters 10 and 11). Depending on the timing, the intensity, duration and extent of this epileptic dysfunction, the behavioral and cognitive regression may be mild and transient (mainly an acquired attention deficit) and more rarely a severe dysexecutive cognitive and behavioral deficit as described above (Deonna 1997). In these instances, a close and direct relationship between acquired behavioral- and cognitive deficits and the epileptic activity is methodologically much more difficult to ascertain than in cases with acquired language deficits, so that this dimension may be underestimated.

In some cases with ECSWS and with an acquired frontal syndrome initially thought to belong to the severest end of the EAS spectrum on the basis of unremarkable early development, electroclinical features and a normal brain MRI, doubt remains that they nevertheless harbor a focal cortical dysplasia or a regional microdysgenesis. The latter can sometimes be found via pathology at follow-up, when seizures relapse after puberty and epilepsy surgery is finally undertaken (Roulet-Perez 1991 and 1998). Follow-up of such children can show persistent epileptiform discharges after remission of seizures and CSWS (Veggiotti 2001; Seegmuller 2012). We thus strongly suspect that in these severe cases, the epilepsy may have a structural aetiology that was missed or escaped current imaging techniques. The link of such cases with the self-limited syndromes of the EAS remains to be further clarified. Recent discoveries in genetics such as the finding that mutations in DEPDC5 which regulates the mTOR pathway can at once be found in familial focal epilepsies without visible lesions (Dibbens et al. 2013; Lal et al. 2015) but also in familial focal epilepsies with focal dysplasia (Baulac 2016) may open new avenues in our understanding.

As mild executive function deficits were recently found in drug naïve children with new-onset typical rolandic epilepsy (Filippini 2016), one can wonder if cortical regions outside the perisylvian network such as the prefrontal cortex may also be involved prior to epilepsy onset as part of a subtle innate brain pathology.

Like patients who present with LKS or AEOS and a history of a specific speech and language impairement prior to epilepsy onset, some children with an IFE or an ECSWS with an acquired frontal syndrome can have a history of a prior attention deficit and mild behavioral disturbances: in these cases, one can speculate that the different clinical picture may be explained by the preferential expression of a basically same innate pathology in the prefrontal rather than perisylvian circuitry, later worsened by the epileptic dysfunction.

Conclusion: the role of epilepsy and/or EEG paroxysmal discharges in rolandic epilepsy

In summary, while the various acquired prolonged and selective reversible cognitive deficits seen sometimes in the course of initially typical rolandic epilepsy described in this section are clearly related to the increased activity of IED (as seen on the EEG, Deonna 2001; Baglietto et al. 2001; Filippini et al. 2013), it is less clear that minor degrees of such impairments also have the same origin. It is especially difficult to disentangle the role of the epilepsy itself from a developmental anomaly when the observed deficits are already present for a long time or only recognized later in the course of development when new skills are not emerging at the expected time, without any notion of a regression. The age at onset of the EEG discharges, their initial and subsequent localizations and spread within the same hemisphere or contralaterally, the degree of activation of IEDs during sleep and the presence of multifocal discharges differ from case to case and in the same child over time. A focal epileptic activity that arises in networks that have completed their maturation or are not participating in cognitive function may cause no harm.

In an individual case, there is often doubt that a moderate or gradual improvement in a specific cognitive domain or in behaviour is really the result IED suppression with an AED. Systematic studies on this issue are fraught with major methodological problems (Pressler et al. 2005 and see Chapter 12). Minor non-specific or behavioural side effects of AEDs may also obscure cognitive improvement due to IED suppression. In rolandic epilepsy, one has to keep in mind that one is not dealing with major cognitive or language regression with a high density of discharges during waking and sleep in which a clinical change under therapy is obvious. Finally, a developmental or an epilepsy-induced permanent structural change in the concerned network may already be present when therapy is started and can limit recovery. Despite all these difficulties, a trial of AEDs in selected cases can be justified (see Chapter 12).

9
LABORATORY INVESTIGATIONS IN LANDAU–KLEFFNER SYNDROME AND THE EPILEPSY-APHASIA SPECTRUM

Electroencephalographic findings

GENERAL FEATURES

Landau–Kleffner syndrome (LKS) as part the EAS spectrum has many characteristics in common with rolandic epilepsy, except that the predominant epileptic focus is located in the posterior temporal rather than the centrotemporal region. The characteristic electroencephalogram (EEG) pattern of rolandic epilepsy is a biphasic spike or a sharp wave followed by a slow wave with a horizontal dipole appearing on a normal background activity in clusters of two or three ('doublets' or 'triplets') and activated by sleep (Pan and Luders 2000). The spikes may be multifocal and independent. The topography, number and extension of these foci can change in the course of the disease ('migrating foci'). Generalized spike waves may also occur usually resulting from bilateral synchrony. Some studies have looked at the EEGs of patients with rolandic epilepsy who subsequently developed LKS or other neuropsychological deficits. Massa et al. (2001) found six interictal EEG patterns predictive of neuropsychological impairments in rolandic epilepsy: One was quantitative, abundance of IED during wakefulness and sleep, and five were qualitative: (1) intermittent slow-wave focus; (2) multiple asynchronous spike-wave foci; (3) long spike-wave clusters; (4) generalized 3c/s 'absence like' spike-wave discharges and (5) conjunction of interictal paroxysms, with negative or positive myoclonia. It remains to be confirmed whether any single or combination of these EEG findings has a predictive value for cognitive deficits early in the course of the disease. A crucial point regarding the EEG abnormalities in LKS is their variability, sometimes correlating with fluctuations in clinical symptoms, both in types and in severity. Sleep activation of the focal interictal epileptiform discharges is a common denominator of the EAS syndromes, but it can be more or less intense, ample, synchronous and diffuse. A CSWS pattern in the narrow sense can be found in LKS, underscoring the overlap with non-lesional ECSWS, but not in all cases. Sleep activation can vary during the same night or from one recording to the other, in terms of intensity and diffusion. Focal spikes may be seen only during sleep in periods of remission. However, spikes tend to occur after the onset of sleep and rarely only later in the night, so that a nap sleep recording is sufficient for routine follow-ups under therapy.

Some children finally diagnosed with LKS had initially a normal sleep EEGs, while they already had a severe language impairment. The best documented cases are described below.

LKS WITH NORMAL EEG RECORDINGS

Van Bogeart et al. (2013) reported three children with profound verbal auditory agnosia in whom a normal sleep EEG (during a nap sleep in two, and a full night sleep in one) was found several months after the onset of language regression. A diagnosis of LKS was made when subsequent sleep EEGs showed focal interictal discharges and CSWS. The authors considered fluctuation of the EEG abnormalities as the most likely explanation mainly because alternation between normal EEG and a CSWS pattern was documented in one case. This represents probably an extreme example of the well-known phenomenon of fluctuating EEG abnormalities previously described in LKS (Aicardi 1986; Hirsch et al. 1990). Another explanation would be that IEDs were not recorded because of sampling limitations (two records with only stage 1 and 2 sleep). These cases imply that a normal sleep EEG does not rule out LKS and that a repeat recording – when possible a whole night – has to be proposed a few weeks after a first negative finding, when there is a strong clinical suspicion of LKS. They also show that language symptoms are not necessarily time locked with the epileptiform activity, and that this has to be explained by any pathophysiological theory (see Chapter 10).

CONTRIBUTION OF PEROPERATIVE ELECTROCORTICOGRAPHY

The localization and extent of the epileptogenic zone in LKS was first convincingly demonstrated by Morrell et al. (1995) on electrocorticography in severe cases before multiple subpial intracortical transsection (MST; Fig 9.1).

Although the epileptogenic zone was mainly found around the sylvian fissure and in the posterior temporal region – on the right side as often as on the left – it also involved, in some cases, parietal and lower frontal regions. Actually, the involved cortical areas corresponded anatomically to those belonging to the language network described in the new model of Hickok and Poeppel (2009, chapter 4).

Corticography was performed on the side of the focus revealed with an intra-carotid injection of a barbiturate. This procedure suppressed the diffuse EEG discharges that reflect propagation from the cortical focus, that is, bilateral synchrony. Currently, computer-aided measures of inter-hemispheric latencies of bilateral discharges are developed to determine the driving hemisphere in pre-surgical work-ups. These seem to be reliable when compared to pharmacological testing and can also be applied to patients with LKS (Martín Miguel et al. 2011).

Corticography naturally cannot provide information about the propagation of the discharges to the controlateral hemisphere or about the presence of a less active independent focus on the other side. Both can happen, as shown several years later by new electrophysiological and functional imaging techniques (see Chapter 11).

MAGNETOENCEPHALOGRAPHY

Studies with magnetoencephalography (MEG) in LKS have further precisely identified the location and spread of the epileptic abnormalities. In Lewine's study of six cases (5 to 9 years) 'sources of primary spikes localized to posterior aspect of the upper bank (opercular

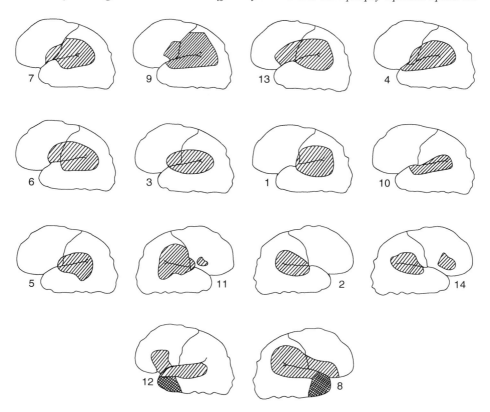

Fig. 9.1. 'Diagrams of the extent of the subpial transsection in 14 patients. Since the subpial transsection was invariably guided by the electrocorticographically defined abnormality, these diagrams also indicate the spatial boundaries of the epileptogenic area'. (Reprinted from Morrell et al., Landau-Kleffner syndrome: Treatment with subpial intracortical transection, *Brain*, 118, 1529–1546, © 1995 Oxford University Press. Used with permission.)

surface) of the superior temporal gyrus, 1 to 3cm deep into the sylvian plane, with additional primary (independant) and /or secondary (propagated) with MEG, involvement of Wernicke's area and the supramarginal gyrus' (Lewine 1999). In 28 children (3y 5m to 12y) with LKS also studied with MEG (2009), Paetau (2009) found bilateral spikes in 12 (42%), unilateral spikes in 4 and no spikes in 3. Independent spikes were found in the sylvian cortex in 2 and outside the sylvian cortex in 3 (parietal, occipital and/or frontal). Of course, different findings can be expected, depending on the moment and severity of the LKS when the recording was carried out, information that was not provided in these studies. MEG in LKS is further discussed in Chapter 11.

Brain imaging

CONVENTIONAL BRAIN MRI

With few exceptions, conventional brain MRI does not show any structural lesion in LKS. Cases of acquired epileptic aphasia due to a structural lesion quoted as 'symptomatic LKS' have already been discussed (see Chapter 2). In most of these, the language deficit resulted from a focal epileptic dysfunction due to a lesion within or close to language areas and clinical and EEG findings were different from non-lesional LKS (see Chapter 2). Focal cortical dysplasias can generate abundant sleep-activated focal IEDs and CSWS, but in this situation, patients often have more seizures than those with an IFE. Nevertheless, rare cases masquerading as typical non-lesional LKS exist (cf. case Huppke, Chapter 2), and it is therefore wise to perform a brain MRI during the initial work-up to rule out any associated pathology, given the potentially prolonged course of the disease and the therapeutic implications. When an abnormality is found by the radiologist, great care has to be taken to interpret it in the clinical context because incidental findings can also occur (Chapter 2).

Since LKS is part of the EAS spectrum including rolandic epilepsy, one also wonders how often MRI abnormalities are present in the latter. In recent years, it has become a routine to perform an MRI in rolandic epilepsy to rule out a lesional epilepsy when clinical or EEG features are atypical or as a criterion for inclusion in research cohorts. Again, with few exceptions (Lundberg et al. 1999) these show normal results (Boxerman et al. 2007). As seen for LKS, there are occasional unexpected findings, such as a focal dysplasia, a polymicrogyria or a white matter lesion that are otherwise neurologically asymptomatic.

Beyond the resolution of conventional MRI
It is increasingly argued that children with LKS or rolandic epilepsy may have a focal or multifocal microdysgenesis that cannot be detected even with modern structural imaging techniques. In that line, recent genetic findings have shown that some genetic mutations implicated in focal 'epilepsy only', such as mutations in *DEPDC5* first demonstrated in familial focal epilepsy with variable foci (Dibbens et al. 2013) may also be associated with focal cortical dysplasias (Scheffer et al. 2014). This opens the possibility that a locally disturbed cytoarchitecture plays indeed a role in some focal epilepsies and that the borders between a lesional and a non-lesional epilepsy may be more tenuous than so far considered.

While clinical MRI studies of patients with LKS and rolandic epilepsy indeed show no lesion, advanced neuroimaging has started to bring out subtle variations in brain morphology in several cortical regions whose significance need to be confirmed (Pardoe et al. 2013) (see Chapter 8).

Regarding LKS more specifically, a recent study performed in a recovered 27-year-old patient with LKS using diffusion-tensor imaging (DTI) fibre tracking suggested altered pathways in the left arcuate fasciculus (Pullens et al. 2015). Of course, one cannot know from this study whether these alterations were congenital, epilepsy-related or reflecting secondary language reorganization. However, it is a start and if this technique, which unlike fMRI requires no active collaboration of the participant, could be used longitudinally and with appropriate controls, it may provide invaluable insights in the pathophysiology of LKS.

Multimodal functional imaging
In the past decade, the use of functional imaging (positron emission tomography, (PET); fMRI) and new electrophysiological techniques (MEG; electrical source imaging, ESI) in patients with epilepsy has advanced our knowledge on the topography and spread of focal

IED. Each of these techniques provides different pieces of information and when combined in the same patient, they can contribute to understand the pathophysiology of the neuropsychological deficits seen in LKS and ECSWS. With regard to PET, it should be emphasized that without an EEG at the time of FDG uptake, results are difficult to interpret. This multimodal approach is described and discussed in Chapter 10.

An example of what this multimodal approach can bring to the study of LKS is taken here from one of their study (de Tiège et al. 2013).

COMBINED METABOLIC AND ELECTROPHYSIOLOGICAL STUDY IN LKS WITH CSWS

The three children studied by de Tiège et al. (2013) were, respectively, 8 years and 2 months, 7 years and 9 months, and 4 years and 9 months old at the time of study. Their cognitive and behavioral impairments (VAA, preserved intelligence with non-verbal IQ, respectively, 75, 109 and 93) had, respectively, started 6 months, 28 months and 16 months previously. Their EEG showed bilateral focal IEDS (T3 and T4; T3 and T4; C3 and C4) in their waking record while during sleep all had CSWS (SWI index of 85%, 81% and 90% at the time of study). [18F]-fluorodeoxyglucose (FDG-PET) scans were obtained during the waking state, while source reconstruction of time-sensitive neurophysiological signals was obtained via magnetic source imaging during induced sleep. The source of the spike-wave discharges was located in the superior temporal gyrus (unilateral: two patients; independent bilateral: one patient), with rapid propagation (5–20ms) towards the contralateral homologue side. Increased glucose metabolism was found on the superior temporal gyrus. It was bilateral in two patients, unilateral on the left side in one patient (patient 3). One of the patients with bilateral increased metabolism also showed significant hypometabolism in the prefrontal cortex (patient 1) (Fig 9.2).

This correlative metabolic and electrophysiological study of these three children with LKS with quite similar symptoms and EEG findings (awake and sleep) and studied in the same active phase of the epilepsy syndrome showed common, but also different findings. They all

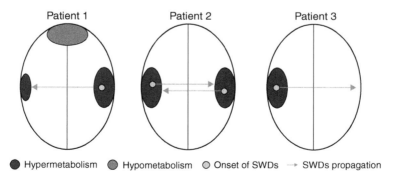

Fig. 9.2. Three patients described in text showing, respectively, bilateral temporal hypermetabolism (dark grey) on FDG-PET in patients 1 and 2 and unilateral left temporal hypermetabolism in patient 3. Patient 1 also had hypometabolism (light grey) in prefrontal cortex. SWDs, spike and wave discharges. Reproduced from De Tiège. et al. Neurophysiological activity underlying altered brain metabolism in epileptic encephalopathies with CSWS. *Epilepsy Res.* 105, 316–325 © 2013, with permission from Elsevier.

had a hypermetabolic focus in the expected superior temporal region corresponding to the focal epileptogenic zone(s), as found in two previous studies (Maquet et al. 1995; Luat et al. 2006). Rapid propagation of the focal interictal discharges from the source to the homologous contralateral area was recorded in all cases. In one case, however, this was not associated with a zone of increased metabolism on the other side. Decreased metabolism in the prefrontal area in patient 1 did not correspond with the source and the propagation zone of the focal discharges, but to more remotely connected areas (See Chapter 11 for further discussion).

These findings are congruent with the notion that either unilateral or bilateral independent epileptic foci occur in LKS, and that contralateral spread from the abnormal electrical activity from the driving side is sufficient to lead to severe and prolonged VAA. Of interest is also that its 'translation' into 'visible' bilateral metabolic changes is not necessarily present.

LKS as an inflammatory or autoimmune epilepsy
An inflammatory aetiology for LKS has been repeatedly suggested and pursued for many years, in view of its remittent- recurrent course and response to corticosteroids or ACTH. However, no consistent evidence of inflammation in CSF or at histology (Chapter 2), of immune deficits or of antibodies to specific brain cells has so far been found. In a very recent patient with refractory LKS who became seizure-free after a right temporo-parietal resection, pathology revealed gliosis, but no abnormality in favour of an inflammation (Fine 2014).

This implies that in a clinical setting, when a child with LKS presents with a typical course and EEG findings, CSF analysis and other searches for an inflammatory or auto-immune disease are not indicated.

In research, the hypothesis of a causal role of inflammation and auto-immunity in LKS and EAS syndromes has been revived because the contribution of these mechanisms to epilepsy in general is increasingly acknowledged (Vezzani et al. 2011 for a review). Several inflammatory mediators such as cytokines (interleukins, interferons, tumour necrosis factors and growth factors) and chemokines can be produced in the CNS by neurons, glial and endothelial cells triggered by an infection, an autoimmune disease or tissue damage. Inflammatory mediators in turn trigger molecular cascades in the neurons and astrocytes that can lead to changes in ion-channels and neurotransmitter receptors activity, neurotransmitter release (mainly glutamate), as well as in neuronal sprouting and synaptogenesis. Cytokines in the CNS can also provoke rupture of the blood brain barrier allowing the passage of peripheral immune cells and mediators. In order to control the potentially dangerous collateral effects of activation of the immune-inflammatory system, nature has provided complex regulatory mechanisms acting at each step of the cascades, among them glucocorticoids (Vezzani 2011). In case of failure of this endogenous control, inflammation results in increased neuronal excitability that can provoke and perpetuate epileptic seizures in a vicious circle. Inflammation can also be the result of epileptic seizures *per se*, regardless of the initial cause. The role of inflammatory mechanisms in triggering and perpetuating epilepsy and the potential preventive and curative effects of anti-inflammatory and immune-modulating drugs are currently an active field of research.

Epileptic seizures are a common feature of autoimmune diseases – systemic or confined to the CNS – and of autoimmune encephalitis in children (Suleiman and Dale 2015). The latter can be focal or diffuse and are usually characterized by an altered level of consciousness, cognition and behaviour, movement disorders and other neurological signs. EEG recordings disclose diffuse or focal slowing, with or without epileptiform activity and seizures. Brain MRI and CSF may be normal. The diagnosis reposes on the findings of specific anti-neuronal autoantibodies in the serum and/or CSF, such as anti-NMDA receptor antibodies (the most frequent in children) and a positive response to immunotherapy. Paediatric cases of sudden-onset epilepsy associated with behavioural and cognitive manifestations, such as those described below, begin to appear in the literature as searches for anti-neuronal antibodies are increasingly carried out.

Cases

This previously typically developing boy presented at the age of 2 years 10 months with a one-year history of daily unprovoked temper tantrums. These lasted a few minutes and were followed by a 10-minute period of sitting quiet and absent-minded. He lost appetite and weight and he became clumsy with slurred speech. Two months later, he developed tonic seizures of one-minute duration with post-ictal sleep and transient expressive language impairment. He had additional headaches and sleep disturbances and the whole clinical picture followed a fluctuating course (Wuerfel et al. 2014). Both his neurological examination and his brain MRI and CSF examination were normal, including oligoclonal bands. The interictal EEG showed multifocal predominantly frontal and right parietal irregular spike and polyspike – waves. At the age of 4 years 5 months, glycine receptor (GlyR) antibodies were found in the boy's serum (but not in CSF) by two renowned laboratories using different techniques. Intravenous methylprednisolone pulse therapy (20mk/kg for 3 days, once monthly) was administered for 6 months, with rapid clinical improvement within 2 months. Seizures and the other symptoms subsided. Six months after the end of therapy, the GlyR antibodies were still measurable, but the titre was lower. Besides, the discussion of the clinical phenotype of GlyR antibody disease, pathogenesis and response to therapy, which are beyond the scope of this book, the authors concluded that, 'This finding points towards a primary phenomenon and possibly pathogenic role of neuronal antibodies in childhood epilepsies with unusual courses as observed here' and 'we encourage the routine investigation of neuronal antibodies in unclassified and therapy refractory epilepsies and fluctuating psychopathological symptoms in childhood.' (Suleiman and Dale 2015).

Some features of this case could suggest an EAS, but the somatic manifestation (headaches and weight loss) as well as the seizure types and EEG findings should urge one to look further than just an 'idiopathic' aetiology.

So far, there is no evidence for a causal role of autoimmunity in EAS and in other non-lesional age-limited focal epilepsies. In a first prospective observational study of a cohort of 114 children with new-onset seizures and classified according to the new proposed ILAE classification of epilepsies and epilepsy syndromes (Suleiman et al. 2013), 11 patients (9.7%) were found to have auto-antibodies to neuronal antigens (VGKC, CASPR2 and NMDAR) compared to 4.6% in controls. Seven had an epilepsy of unknown cause, which was focal in four cases. None had an epilepsy or EEG findings compatible with an IFE or EAS.

To our knowledge, the studies suggesting the presence of various 'anti-brain' autoantibodies in some patients with LKS, ECSWS and atypical rolandic epilepsy (Boscolo et al. 2005; Connolly et al. 2006) were not replicated. It is possible that new discoveries will be made in this field with the more widespread use of anti-neuronal antibodies panels and new methods to assess immune mediators, but there is still a long way to go. At this stage, one has to warn against taking the striking effect of corticosteroids or ACTH on the sleep-activated IED in LKS as evidence of an inflammatory or autoimmune aetiology. This drug effect is also observed in epilepsy with continuous spikes and waves during sleep associated with various brain lesions in which there is so far no evidence of autoimmunity, and many other biological effects of these hormones may explain their antiepileptic action.

Genetics of EAS

CLINICAL GENETIC STUDIES

From the first publications on LKS, familial cases have been described. There was one sibling pair in Landau and Kleffner's original article (1957), one sibling pair in Worster–Drought series (1971) and one in Rapin's cases of VAA (1977). It is noteworthy that one patient of this latter study has had a daughter with rolandic epilepsy (Rapin, pers. comm. 2012). However, the fact that most cases of LKS seem to be sporadic and that an identical twin pair was found discordant for LKS (Feekery et al. 1993) has casted doubt on the importance of genetic factors in LKS (Conroy et al. 2014).

This doubt was reinforced by a study looking at twins with rolandic epilepsy (Vadlamudi et al. 2006): Among 18 twin pairs (10 monozygous, 8 dizygous) with typical rolandic epilepsy, none was found to be concordant for rolandic epilepsy and none had seizures (1 uncertain). Concordance for centro-temporal spikes was documented in one monozygous twin pair only. The authors who belong to a renowned Australian group focusing on the genetics of epilepsies (Vadlamudi et al. 2006) concluded that their own findings challenged the role of genetic factors in typical rolandic epilepsy.

Looking at the issue with a different angle, the same group (Vears et al. 2012) and Tsai (2013) scrutinized the family history of seizures in the spectrum of IFE, including LKS, typical rolandic epilepsy and related cases. In Tsai et al.'s study, 31 children belonging to the EAS were recruited according to defined electro-clinical criteria (sleep activation pattern, seizure types and cognitive profile). Children with LKS ($n = 3$), ESCWS ($n = 5$) and atypical benign partial epilepsy ($n = 1$) were included as well as a new subgroup called 'intermediate aphasia epilepsy disorders' (IAED) ($n = 22$). The latter comprised children 'with cognitive regression, delay, or plateauing (predominantly in the language domain) with centrotemporal epileptiform discharges that showed sleep activation yet did not fulfil the criteria for CSWS' (Tsai et al. 2013). Children with typical rolandic epilepsy, those with tonic seizures or those with seizure and cognitive manifestations but a normal EEG, were excluded. The authors analysed the seizure history, looking at first-, second- and third-degree relatives, via a detailed questionnaire and evaluated the frequency and the phenotype of the epilepsy in these relatives. Among the 31 probands, 16 (51.6%) has a family history of seizures and among all relatives ($N = 1254$) 30 (2.4%) had seizures, including 19 (1.5%) with epilepsy and 13 (1%) with febrile seizures (2 having both). Of the 19 relatives with epilepsy, only 4 had rolandic epilepsy and 3 IEAD (1 monozygous twin pair). The others had either focal epilepsy of unknown cause (4), genetic generalized epilepsy (1) or unclassified epilepsy (1). In several families, different family phenotypes could be found (e.g. three siblings, respectively, had ECSWS, IEAD and focal epilepsy). Furthermore, and this was the crux of the matter, the EAS cohort was compared with a previously published cohort of children with typical rolandic epilepsy in which a same family search was also performed (Vears et al. 2012). The proportion of probands with a positive family history of seizures was similar in the EAS and rolandic epilepsy cohort as well as the proportion of affected relatives (in total and for each degree of relatedness). The authors concluded that EAS and rolandic epilepsy were on a same clinical continuum and likely to share common genetic determinants These findings are in concordance with the observations from longitudinal studies in which the same child's condition can evolve from one syndrome to another (see Chapter 7). The pattern of seizure inheritance was found to be complex with the probable contribution of multiple genes of small effect and environmental factors in most families. In some families, however, single genes of major effects could play a role.

THE *GRIN2A* SAGA AND CONTRIBUTION OF MOLECULAR GENETIC STUDIES
The use of chromosome microarray testing that can detect copy number variants (CNVs) – that is, small (up to about 50kb) deletions or duplications of chromosomal regions – in patients with intellectual disabilities put clinicians on a new track in the genetics of LKS and ECSWS. In 2010, a microdeletion in the 16p13 region was found in three unrelated patients with intellectual disability (absent speech in 2/3), dysmorphic features and rolandic seizures but no visible brain malformation (Reutlinger et al. 2010). The authors were able to target the critical region for the epilepsy phenotype to *GRIN2A*. This gene was a suitable candidate because it encodes the NR2A subunit of the NMDA receptor, a glutamate-gated ion channel. *GRIN2A* was previously singled-out as a candidate gene in autistic spectrum disorder (Barnby et al. 2005) and in familial or sporadic intellectual disability with various types of epilepsies (Endele et al. 2010). One family in the latter small series included two affected members with bilateral centro-temporal spikes, activated by sleep in one, without seizures. The detection of a *de novo* partial deletion in *GRIN2A* in a case of LKS from a cohort of 61 patients ECSWS or LKS (Lesca et al. 2013) was a further prompt to look more deeply into the role of this gene in the rolandic epilepsy spectrum. This was simultaneously achieved in 2013 by three groups (Lesca et al. 2013; Lemke et al. 2013; Carvill et al. 2013), which found *GRIN2A* mutations in 9%–20% of three different cohorts of patients (including familial cases) with LKS, ECSWS, APBE and other atypical forms of rolandic epilepsy, and in 3.6% (13/358) of those with typical rolandic epilepsy (Turner et al. 2015a, b). All probands with 4 GRIN2A mutations from Carvill et al. (2013) were familial cases and Lesca et al. (2013) also found 10 affected families. From the epilepsy viewpoint, affected members of a same family either had the same epilepsy syndrome (ECSWS, atypical rolandic epilepsy) or a different one (CSWS, LKS and atypical rolandic epilepsy in one large three generations family). Not all individuals with mutations appeared to have epilepsy and some had febrile seizures only (see Table 1 in Turner et al. 2015b for a detailed review of the epilepsy phenotype in individuals with *GRIN2A*-mutations). It is noteworthy that

family A in Carvill et al. (2013) was the family with autosomal dominant rolandic epilepsy and speech dyspraxia (ADRESD) initially reported by Scheffer et al. (1995), and that this family shared the same mutation and haplotypes with their family C, so that they probably had a common ancestor, unknown to them (Turner et al. 2015b). Their speech and language phenotype was quite similar (see below) as well as their seizure type (rolandic), but the main EEG features were sleep-activated CTS in family A and multifocal, in addition to more posterior discharges with CSWS in family B.

In the three cohorts of patients (Lesca et al. 2013; Lemke et al. 2013; Carvill 2013), individuals with *GRIN2A*-mutations were reported to have either normal or delayed early development (globally or in the speech and language domain). In a same family (family D, Carvill et al. 2013), affected individuals had normal or delayed early milestones (between generations and within the same generation). Regarding the cognitive phenotype, intelligence was considered normal or mildly impaired, and a few patients had autistic traits in a context of global intellectual deficit (Lesca et al. 2013). The terms 'verbal dyspraxia', 'dysphasia with impaired speech production' and 'dysphasia' not otherwise specified were often used.

Three families (A, C and D) from Carvill et al. (2013) including the princeps ADRESD family were studied in details by Turner et al. (2015b). Eleven members with mutations had a strikingly similar phenotype of oromotor and speech difficulties consisting in poorly coordinated lip and tongue movements, dysarthria and speech dyspraxia with altered prosody. These features were sometimes quite subtle and severity was variable within the same family. Language and intelligence were impaired in some but not in all patients; none had VAA. Speech disturbances were reported before seizure onset in most and persisted after the disappearance of the epileptiform abnormalities. They also occurred in two individuals with mutations without a seizure history, and this was also reported in two families in Lesca et al.'s study (2013). Turner et al. (2015b) hence concluded that the speech and language impairment were unlikely to be due to the epileptiform activity and that *GRIN2A* may play a role in normal speech production. However, since epileptiform activity can precede seizure onset and have a deleterious impact on speech and language development, this statement remains to be further confirmed, the more so that some patients had early seizure onset (between 1 year and 5 months and 2 years and 5 months). The observation that some patients had language and cognitive regression (Family C and D, Carvill et al. 2013) and that impairments were more severe in the younger patients (< 21years) who had ECSWS and IEAD (Turner et al. 2015a) indicates that the epilepsy played an additional role.

In our opinion, the consequences of a modified NMDA receptor activity on the development of speech/language, motor and more global-learning capacities in infants independently from the epilepsy remain unsettled. It seems unlikely that *GRIN2A* will turn out to be a key player in typical rolandic epilepsy, but it establishes a 'molecular link' between the EAS. Its place in developmental speech and language disorders without epilepsy is not known yet. One can postulate that the development and excitability of the speech production networks may be preferentially affected by *GRIN2A* mutations. It is not yet clear if such mutations have been found in patients with VAA 'only'. The epilepsy can cause a specific either novel or additional dysfunction to a previous congenital delay: it will consist of a speech and language regression if it remains confined to the perisylvian networks and a more global deterioration if diffuse CSWS are generated, with effects on more remote cognitive networks (see Chapter 9).

In another genetic study, Conroy et al. (2014) used a multi-faceted approach combining comparative genomic hybridisation (CGH), whole genome methylation profiling and exome sequencing in a cohort of 13 patients with LKS – 11 isolated cases and 2 pairs of discordant monozygotic (MZ) twins, including that of Feekery et al. (1993). Besides one *GRIN2A* mutation, they found no single other but a number of additional interesting candidate genes, including *RELN*, *BSN*, *EPHB2* and *NID2*. The clinical discordance between the MZ twin pairs could not be explained by discordant CNVs or discordant methylation. Somatic mosaïcism was not assessed. The authors proposed that genetic variants may be at the origin of LKS, but that additional environmental factors and structural abnormalities contribute to render the genetic susceptibility clinically manifest.

The recent review by Turner et al. (2015b) provides a table of inherited and de novo CNVs that may be relevant in AES.

Genetic investigations in IFE still have a long way to go. For the clinician faced with an individual case of EAS, the finding of one or the other of the reported genetic abnormality or variant has to be interpreted carefully. A negative finding does not discard a genetic aetiology, nor indicates that exogenous factors are the main cause of the epilepsy syndrome.

10
PHYSIOPATHOLOGY OF SPEECH, LANGUAGE AND OTHER PROLONGED EPILEPTIC DYSFUNCTION IN LANDAU–KLEFFNER SYNDROME, EPILEPSY WITH CONTINUOUS SPIKE WAVES DURING SLEEP AND RELATED SYNDROMES

Introduction

The effects of a focal epileptic activity originating in a cortical region or in a particular set of neurons that are part of a cognitive network (i.e. interacting neural circuits supporting a cognitive function) will depend on the consequences of the bioelectrical changes (excitation/inhibition) it induces locally and more remotely by propagation via established short- and long-distance connections (cf. Chapter 11). Impact on cognition can be limited when the concerned network underpins a localized and modular skill (e.g. visual or auditory perception and graphomotor skill) or more pervasive when the affected circuits are the substrate of more complex and widely distributed processes (attention and memory consolidation) (see Fig 10.1). In addition to the epilepsy-induced dysfunction that can be circumscribed, one has to take into account the downstream effect of the loss of a given function on those depending on it, which can be considerable. This is best illustrated by verbal auditory agnosia in which a localized dysfunction in the auditory cortices will interfere not only with the patients' speech comprehension but also its expression by interrupting the auditory feedback from his own production.

While the variable dynamics of the installation and course of the aphasia in LKS can readily be accepted as an argument in favour of its epileptic origin, the absence of immediate correlation with the electroencephalogram (EEG) findings and the long-term sequelae are often taken against it.

Table 10.1 summarizes the dynamics of evolution observed in patients diagnosed with LKS from the first symptoms and through the course of the disease until the final stage. This is essentially its natural course, although therapy can modify it for the better or the worse. It is noteworthy that the same child can have episodes of acute, subacute or slow onset and recovery, with variable degree of severity at different periods.

TABLE 10.1
Dynamics of language deficit in Landau-Kleffner syndrome

Acute versus insidious slow onset

Acute onset then slow aggravation (or reverse)

Rapid versus slow recovery

No recovery

Monophasic versus relapsing – remitting course

Note: These variable patterns can be seen in different patients or in the same child at different periods of the disease, months or years apart.

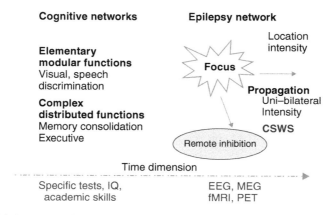

Fig. 10.1. Link between epilepsy and cognitive networks. Specific neuropsychological tools are needed to assess elementary localized modular and more complex distributed functions. Multimodal techniques can help better define where and how the epileptic and cognitive networks overlap.

Morrell et al. (1995) were the first to perform electro-corticographic studies in a few children with severe LKS who were considered for epilepsy surgery (see Chapters 2 and 9). These studies demonstrated that the continuous diffuse epileptic discharges were driven by an epileptic focus located in the perisylvian region. One of the authors (TD) had the privilege to read the original clinical notes on the first 2 of the 14 children who underwent MST. Language improvement did not immediately follow cessation of the IEDs but was gradual over several months, so that the direct role of the epilepsy was questioned. These effects of surgery were difficult to interpret but certainly confirmed that there was no simple relation between the IED and the aphasia, at least when it was severe and prolonged.

Pathophysiology of the acquired epileptic aphasia in LKS
This chapter reviews the clinical and electrophysiological data that have been adduced to support a direct role of epilepsy in the acquired aphasia in LKS. One must acknowledge that the 'epileptic aphasia' seen in LKS does not fit well the classical ictal-post-ictal cognitive deficits seen in other epilepsies, but it is necessary to start from that point.

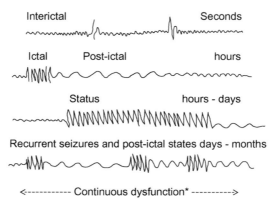

Fig. 10.2. Duration of temporary cognitive dysfunction in correlation with EEG epileptic activity. Classic models. From Deonna T and Roulet-Perez E. Cognitive and Behavioural Disorders of Epileptic Origin in Children. Clinics in Developmental Medicine No. 168. London; Mac Keith Press, 2005, p11.

Figure 10.2 illustrates the types of deficits – here cognitive – that can be directly correlated with the epileptic activity recorded on the EEG.

The first and briefest deficit is the so-called transient cognitive impairment (TCI) meaning that the epileptiform discharges interfere directly with ongoing cognitive processing such as attending, encoding, retrieving and responding to a stimulus that may be task specific (Aarts et al. 1984, Pressler and Brandl 1995).

The second is a cognitive deficit as the main manifestation of the seizure itself or of a post-ictal deficit, like, for instance, ictal or post-ictal aphasia. The latter can be seen as an equivalent of Todd's paresis due to active surround inhibition and lasts for a variable period. If the seizure itself is prolonged (status epilepticus), there will be a corresponding functional impairment usually followed by a reversible but sometimes permanent post-ictal deficit.

If seizures that are not always clinically obvious occur frequently, there is no time for recovery between them and the deficit will appear continuous and long lasting.

In EAS/LKS, the prolonged deficits most often have no clear-cut clinical–EEG correlates and no relationship with periods of frequent seizures (actually some patients never had any). They are thus, not explained by this classic model.

For instance, the 'on-line' suppression of EEG discharges with antiepileptic drugs under EEG monitoring does not bring language back immediately or within hours, as one can see in cases of ictal aphasias.

Language recovery is seen after the EEG has improved or normalized, but this occurs more often over days, weeks or months rather than hours. For such cases of slow onset, prolonged deficits without seizures but related to abundant often markedly sleep-activated 'interictal' discharges, the term 'paraictal' deficit has been proposed (Shafrir and Prensky 1995) and a functional inhibition in and around the concerned epileptogenic zone is postulated.

Regarding permanent sequelae, it is assumed that epileptiform discharges occurring for a prolonged period in an immature brain can modify and alter the developing neuronal cells and their connectivity in the involved networks. While this has been demonstrated in experimental models of early focal epilepsy, it can only be suspected in LKS (Morrell et al. 1995).

Bilateral reduction of superior temporal regions found via brain volume analysis on MRI in four cases of LKS (Takeoka et al. 2004) suggests epilepsy-induced damage, but one cannot prove that these changes were acquired and not congenital because the patients were only studied once. Functional imaging studies done at various stages in the evolution of LKS and other focal epilepsy syndromes with continous spike waves during slow sleep (CSWS) are giving new indirect evidence for acquired persistent or permanent dysfunction locally or at distance from the original epileptic focus (see Chapter 11).

Actually, it is more likely that a variable combination of the above-discussed mechanisms explains the acquired cognitive and motor deficits observed in LKS and other EASs. Children with rolandic epilepsy who present with acquired prolonged, albeit reversible oromotor and speech deficits, that is, the acquired anterior epileptic opercular syndrome (AEOS; see Chapter 8) are suggestive of such combined mechanisms. The pathophysiology of AEOS can be assumed to be the same as in LKS, although affecting another part of the language networks, with the advantage that oromotor and expressive speech deficits are clinically more obvious and easier to correlate with EEG findings than with receptive deficits. A review of the rare correlative clinical-EEG and functional imaging studies of these cases is therefore in place here.

Acquired epileptic opercular syndrome: a combination of ictal-post-ictal and 'paraictal' oromotor and speech deficits (Table 10.2)

The coining of the term 'acquired epileptic opercular syndrome' (Shafrir and Prensky 1995; see Chapter 8) provided a wider recognition of a subset of children who present with acquired prolonged but reversible oromotor and speech deficits and a fluctuating course. The EEG discloses high amplitude centro-temporal discharges that become bilateral and activated by sleep, whether meeting or not the criteria of CSWS.

In addition to drooling, oromotor dysfunction and dysarthria, some of these children have frequent rolandic seizures as well as brief myoclonic jerks of the face or limbs. These can provoke falls or weakness or motor neglect of the affected body part when frequent (Paquier et al. 2009). On the EEG of these children, the bilateral or diffuse-spike discharges dominant in the rolandic regions become synchronous with hemifacial twitching and may be inhibited by voluntary mouth and tongue movements (Gobbi et al. 2006). These jerks can correspond to a phenomenon called 'epileptic negative myoclonus', that is, a sudden, brief (< 500ms) interruption of tonic muscle activity on the electromyogram (EMG) without the contraction of the agonist–antagonists muscles seen in 'positive myoclonia' (see Rubboli and Tassinari 2006 for review). Negative myoclonus seems to be related to a negative component of the spike occurring just before the slow wave or with the slow wave itself (Rubboli and Tassinari 2006).

In the child with rolandic epilepsy and three phases of AEOS studied by de Saint-Martin et al. (1999), uni-or bilateral independent facial myoclonia involving the corner of the mouth, the inferior lip and the eye lid were observed (see Chapter 8). These were either isolated or occurred in clusters at a frequency of several per minutes to a few per day. According to the authors, 'image-by-image video-EEG confrontation revealed that single

TABLE 10.2
Summary of epilepsy-related manifestations in acquired epileptic opercular syndrome

Frequent rolandic seizures with transient post-ictal deficit: facial weakness, 'speech arrest' and or other speech or oromotor deficits.

Rolandic 'status epilepticus': prolonged oromotor and speech deficits with positive or negative myoconic jerks in peribuccal region (sometimes limbs/trunk) associated with continuous bilateral rolandic discharges, but not rolandic seizure pattern. Myoclonic jerks time locked with spike or slow wave.

Isolated prolonged oromotor deficits (days, weeks, months): similar deficit also associated with abundant bilateral centro-temporal IEDS. CSWS are often present, rolandic seizures not necessarily.

IEDS: interictal epileptiform discharges; CSWS: continuous spike waves during slow sleep.

and rhythmic facial myoclonias were always associated with the spike components of contralateral, isolated or repetitive, "interictal" rolandic spike-wave complexes. However, the majority of interictal discharges remained asymptomatic'. Symptomatic discharges differed from asymptomatic ones only by the amplitude of the spike and of the slow wave, especially under the central electrodes. The authors emphasize that these repetitive focal jerks were often referred to in the literature as rolandic 'status epilepticus', but that the corresponding EEG recordings (including in their own case) never revealed the typical ictal pattern of rolandic seizures (focal rhythmical polyspikes and sharp-wave discharges). They concluded, therefore, that in rolandic epilepsy 'interictal spike-wave complexes may directly induce brief opercular symptoms, which are either "positive" and produced by excessive excitation related to the spike components, or "negative" and produced by excessive inhibition associated with slow-wave components'. Longer lasting oromotor and speech deficits also correlated with the amount of bilateral centro-temporal epileptiform discharges but did not occur during or after repeated seizures, so that they did not represent ictal or post-ictal manifestations either. It is noteworthy that in this case increased glucose metabolism was found in both opercular regions via fluoro-desoxy-glucose-positron emission tomography during an active period: focal hypermetabolism is also a hallmark of ECSWS, but not of classic rolandic epilepsy, suggesting a common underlying pathophysiology for, respectively, motor deficit in AEOS and cognitive deficits in LKS/ECSWS (see Chapter 11).

Focal spike-induced cerebral dysfunction

Shewmon and Erwin's (1989) pioneer study documented the effect of posterior focal interictal discharges on visual perception and reaction time in three participants. He showed that the reaction time was prolonged and the non-response rate increased when the stimulus (flash) was presented at the end of the slow wave and not otherwise. The authors concluded that 'the after-coming slow wave (surround hyperpolarization) transiently disrupts aspects of cortical functioning, in addition to whatever effect the spike itself may have. Focal spike-wave induced cortical dysfunction may be relevant to a variety of interictal cognitive disorders'. With the same patients, by varying the side of visual stimulation and hand response, they were also able to show that the maximal spike related focal dysfunction corresponded to its location (Shewmon and Erwin 1988, 1989). The cases were of course adults who did not have IFEs with a majority of interictal discharges during sleep and the stimulus/response was elementary (flash motor response to perception). However, Shewmon's work showed that focal epileptiform discharges may have an 'on-line' impact on specific cerebral functions.

When looking at the difficulty of the experimental protocol and patient's cooperation such a study requires, it is not surprising that this approach is difficult to apply to children with LKS. In order to investigate a possible direct effect of interictal discharges on language processing in the acute and severe phase of LKS, the child needs to be attentive enough during several minutes at least, and has to be explained the task while his comprehension is limited. As previously discussed, short-term variations in comprehension or expression are clinically likely and are sometimes mentioned by parents, especially in recent onset and mild cases. It is, however, uncertain whether this reflects transient spike-related fluctuations of function at the level of a specific neuronal network. Shemon and Erwin's study and few others on TCI in cases of IFE (Kasteliejn et al. 1990 a, b; Binnie 1991, 1992; Pressler and Brandl 1995) with frequent EEG discharges represent the basis of the postulate that 'inter-ictal' discharges may have a deleterious impact justifying clinical drug trials (see Chapter 11; Verrotti et al. 2013 for a review on TCI in rolandic epilepsy).

'On-line' spike-induced auditory processing disturbance in LKS

Only a few attempts to demonstrate how the processing of speech sounds can be directly affected by the epileptic spikes are to be found in the literature.

Seri et al. (1998) recorded spike-triggered auditory evoked responses (to 1kHZ, 40 ms pure tone, at an intensity of 80db bilaterally) in six children with active LKS. The authors concluded that

> left hemisphere spikes are associated with a greater reduction in amplitude and an increase in latency of the N1. (N1 is a large, negative cortical evoked potential that peaks in adults between 80 and 120 milliseconds after the onset of a stimulus. It is elicited by any unpredictable stimulus in the absence of task demands. It is often referred to with the following P200 evoked potential as the "N1-P2" complex.) This increase in latency was more marked with spikes in the left rather than with spikes occurring in the right hemisphere. No stable change in the evoked response was detected outside of the EEG paroxysm.

The authors postulated that 'interictal activity is able to induce impairment in processing auditory information' and that 'this may play a role in the pathogenesis of language deficit in AEA'.

This study has been influential in the thinking that a time-locked alteration of a specific elementary auditory stimulus occurs during the spike-slow wave complex in LKS. Surprisingly, no similar study has been done since, except the one of Boyd et al. (1996) obtained in different conditions and with a divergent conclusion.

A 7-year-old child with global aphasia and severe behavioural disturbances underwent multiple subpial transection (MST). While on general anaesthesia, event-related potentials (ERP) to the phonemes /ba/ and /ga/ were recorded during electrocorticography before the procedure. The ERPs were distributed 'over the middle and inferior temporal gyri and there was a marked overlap with the area of maximal spiking detected on the electrocorticogram'.

Repetition of the frequent syllable /ba/ was associated with diminution of the prominent negative component of the prominent negative of the ERP culminating around 550ms suggesting habituation. Presentation of the novel syllable /ga/ restored the amplitude of this negative component showing that discrimination was preserved despite the global aphasia. Single tones did not evoke spikes. The authors concluded that 'while our findings support the concept of a close association between the epileptogenic zone and cortical areas involved in language-related processing in LKS, they also suggest that the relationship may not be simply one of inhibition of functional cortex by spiking' and that 'These findings support clinical evidence that some children with epileptic aphasia can still process auditory speech input'.

From the data and the scheme provided by the authors, the maximal epileptic activity was found over the left middle temporal sulcus and above the sylvian fissure, close to the lower rolandic area. Of interest is that the child presented with an acute speech disturbance after status epilepticus with subsequent deterioration, so that he became unable to feed himself and to respond to his name. He became aggressive and unmanageable. Responses to environmental sounds were not mentioned. This picture suggests global aphasia with oromotor and speech impairment and possible pre-frontal involvement and not VAA. Preserved speech sound discrimination is perhaps explained here by the fact that the focal epileptic activity actually spared its specific underlying network (especially the auditory cortices) even if there was an overlap of the spiking and the evoked-potentials recording sites on corticography. If the child had had true VAA, the findings could possibly have been other, similar to Seri's cases.

CSWS and their role in language and other types of cognitive–behavioural regression

Since the initial recognition of 'electrical status epilepticus during sleep' (ESES) (Patry et al. 1971), later called CSWS, a number of its characteristics have been gradually delineated (see Chapter 3). These are summarized in Table 10.3.

CSWS: IS THE THALAMUS A KEY PLAYER?

The CSWS pattern can be seen in lesional and non-lesional epilepsies. It is unclear what makes sleep activation of interictal discharges so prominent in some focal epilepsies. Our clinical observation that an early isolated lesion in the thalamus could have a direct role in generating CSWS (Monteiro et al. 2001) has been amply replicated thereafter. In several publications however, the thalamic involvement was part of more extensive brain damage, typically perinatal middle cerebral artery infarcts (Guzzetta et al. 2005; Sánchez-Fernández 2012b). A recent study (Kersbergen et al. 2013) of 14 infants with isolated neonatal thalamic haemorrhage due to cerebral venous sinus thrombosis has confirmed the high incidence of epilepsy (64%) and of 'sleep aggravated epileptiform EEG activity' (three cases of classical CSWS, 2 with 50%–85% of sleep activation, two with 25%–50% activation) in this population. Brain MRIs performed in later childhood in 10 participants showed a residual thalamic lesion in all, with additional small areas of gliosis at the sites of punctate lesions distributed in the white matter seen during the neonatal period in eight of them. It is interesting to see that the pioneer case of de Tiège et al. (2007) had the same MRI findings.

TABLE 10.3
Continuous spike waves during slow sleep pattern: main characteristics

Onset during early-mid childhood

Occurs in non-lesional (idiopathic/genetic) and lesional epilepsies

Can be suppressed by diazepines and steroids but facilitated or provoked by some antiepileptic drugs (carbamazepine) ....

Due to bilateral synchrony (one or more foci, not always evident)

Thalamic nuclei (esp. reticular nucleus) may play a role in their generation

Often associated with cognitive/behavioural regression (variable patterns and courses)

Adapted from Deonna T and Roulet-Perez E. Cognitive and Behavioural Disorders of Epileptic Origin in Children. Clinics in Developmental Medicine No. 168. London; Mac Keith Press, 2005.

In an attempt to identify the thalamic structures generating CSWS, Losito et al. (2015) looked more precisely at the location of thalamic damage in 60 patients with thalamic lesions (only 1 with an isolated lesion) and sleep-activated IED: most patients had unilateral lesions ($n = 44$) with damage in the ventral nuclei including the reticular nucleus ($n = 45$) and in the medial nuclei, including the medio-dorsal nucleus ($n = 27$). An imbalance between the activity of the reticular nucleus containing GABAergic neurons and the medio-dorsal nucleus containing glutaminergic thalamocortical neurons was postulated to play a role in the generation of sleep-activated IEDs (Losito et al. 2015). The authors therefore looked for a correlation between damage in these structures and the magnitude of sleep activation. Involvement of the medio-dorsal nucleus was more frequent (62%) in patients with CSWS (> 85% of sleep) than in those with a lesser degree of sleep activation (37% when sleep activation was 50%–80%, 0% when sleep activation was 10%–50%). The reticular nucleus was involved in most cases (63%–83%), regardless of the degree of sleep activation.

Clinical data converge thus to indicate that injury of the thalamic nuclei can trigger CSWS. Unfortunately, there is no animal model of epilepsy with CSWS. However, the question of whether an early thalamic lesion or dysfunction is alone sufficient to allow CSWS to develop or whether an additional lesion or epileptic focus in the cortex is necessary to trigger the cortico-thalamic circuitry remains unsolved. Uni- or bilateral epileptic foci in various locations are often described in children with early thalamic lesions (Kersbergen et al. 2013; Losito et al. 2015). These could be due either to associated lesions (related to the mechanism that caused the thalamic damage or to the underlying condition - for instance periventricular leukomalacia of prematurity (De Grandis et al. 2014) or induced by the abnormal thalamic activity itself or due to some unrelated genetic predisposition. In any case, their precise role in the generation of the CSWS pattern seen in thalamic damage is unknown. The cat in which there is already experience with thalamic lesions generating spike-wave complexes (Steriade and Contreras 1998; Monteiro et al. 2001) could be a good model in terms of size and differentiation of thalamic nuclei and cortex for studying CSWS during brain maturation and the respective role of each component of the circuitry (Issa 2014).

The contribution of a thalamic dysfunction in children with 'idiopathic' ECSWS and syndromes belonging to the EAS is unknown yet. As with thalamic lesions, an imbalance between GABAergic and glutaminergic neurotransmission in the thalamocortical circuitry due to mutations in relevant genes such as *GRIN2A* may be speculated and studied with animal models (see Chapter 9 on genetics).

CSWS: THEIR ROLE IN LANGUAGE AND OTHER TYPES OF COGNITIVE-BEHAVIOURAL DETERIORATION
Cognitive and behavioural impairments were noted in all children in whom ESES/CSWS were first described (Patry et al. 1971) and were not explained by frequent seizures or underlying lesions. These were often acquired during the course of the epilepsy leading to the hypothesis that CSWS could be at their origin. However, this causal link is questioned until now because the CSWS pattern has no immediate clinical correlate (the children appear to sleep normally) and its time correlation with the cognitive deficits is often difficult to establish (Tassinari et al. 2000; Scholtes et al. 2005; Nickels and Wirrell 2008; Segmuller 2012). Reasons for that are that CSWS are usually already found on the first sleep record and that they can vary over time. In addition, one can occasionally see children with epilepsy who have a CSWS pattern without evident behavioural or cognitive disturbances. Finally, CSWS can disappear without obvious clinical improvement or can reappear without relapse of the neuropsychological deficits. However, when the disease course is considered with a broader time scale, a correlation between CSWS and cognitive deficits is good. This has now been shown in several longitudinal studies (Boel and Casaer 1989). This implies that the impact of CSWS on cognition and behaviour cannot be conceived as a 'status epilepticus' in the sense of the usual definition (cf. Chapter 3) and that other explanations have to be found.

Many factors (age, duration, intensity, location of the driving focus and response to antiepileptic medication) were gradually recognized to influence the nature and severity of the associated neuropsychological deficits.

One way to assess the direct impact of CSWS on cognitive functions is to look at the rare situations in which the children were followed closely before and after these were medically or surgically suppressed.

In a personal observation (Kallay et al. 2009), a boy with a congenital hemiplegia due to an infarct of the medial cerebral artery and a marked global regression (agitation, mutism and aberrant behaviour) with CSWS underwent hemispherotomy at the age of 5 years and 4 months. He remarkably improved in his behaviour within days and cognitively within weeks after surgery. The pre- and post-operative EEG recordings revealed that the CSWS driven by the peri-lesional foci were immediately interrupted by the procedure. The CSWS activity, especially their spread to both 'healthy' frontal regions, was held responsible for the regression. Later, gradual but incomplete recovery was attributed to possible 'structural effects of prolonged epileptic discharges in rapidly developing cerebral networks which are, at the same time, undergoing the reorganization imposed by unilateral early hemispheric lesion' (Kallay et al. 2009). Battaglia et al. (2009) reported a similar case of a child with epilepsy due to a perinatal stroke submitted to hemispherotomy. The clinical evaluation and comparative tests over a short period (one month) showed marked improvement coincident with the cessation of CSWS.

A new source of information about the correlation between CSWS and neuropsychological-behavioural impairment is now becoming available with the recognition of the previously discussed group of children with neonatal thalamic haemorrhage in whom CSWS have a high probability to develop (Kersbergen et al. 2013). In their retrospective study, Kersbergen observed significant differences in development between patients who did have CSWS versus those who did not or had lesser degrees of sleep activation, while the extent of the thalamic lesion appeared the same. Children were treated with various AEDs with mixed results. The authors concluded to a deleterious role of CSWS, although 'a reliable relation between the onset of EEG abnormalities in sleep and the first signs of neurodevelopmental delay was not possible, as sleep EEGS were not always performed early (and serially) in the course of neurodevelopment'. A prospective study of such children would be an opportunity to see which neuropsychological profiles emerge according to the presence (or absence) of associated epileptic foci and their location. To our knowledge, no patient with an isolated thalamic lesion and CSWS was reported to have an acquired epileptic aphasia, but a severe acquired attention and executive deficit with failure to learn was reported in a single case of 'pure' neonatal thalamic haemorrhage due to vitamin K deficiency. This was followed longitudinally by our group from the time ECSWS was diagnosed at 3 years 4 months after normal early development (Gubser-Mercati et al. 2005).

THE ROLE OF CSWS IN THE LANGUAGE DEFICIT OF LKS

The respective role of the focal IEDS versus diffuse sleep activated epileptiform discharges (CSWS) in determining the type of cognitive deficit, here the aphasia, maintaining it and preventing recovery is still an issue that needs to be clarified.

Children with incipient LKS and minor language deficits usually already have sleep activated focal IEDs. When the deficit worsens, these IEDs can become more diffuse and further increase so that their density meet the criteria of CSWS (see Chapter 3). This has created confusion in thinking that the CSWS themselves are the direct and immediate cause of the language impairment. However, it is clear that acquired aphasia can also occur without CSWS, for instance with only focal and unilateral sleep activated IEDs. In fact, there are many cases of LKS who never develop CSWS and if so, only late in the course and when the symptomatology is at its peak. Conversely, patients with ECSWS can have cognitive impairments with preserved language-for instance those with an acquired frontal syndrome (cf. Chapter 6). This clearly shows that CSWS are neither necessary nor sufficient to account for the language symptoms of LKS (Roulet-Perez 1995).

In order to advance this issue, the multimodal electrophysiological and functional imaging approach proposed by De Tiège and Van Bogaert (Chapter 11) that could be applied prospectively to different subsets of children with epilepsies in the EAS appears promising.

DISTURBANCES OF SYNAPTIC HOMEOSTASIS: IS IT A POSSIBLE CAUSE OF NEUROPSYCHOLOGICAL IMPAIRMENT IN ECSWS AND LKS?

Tononi and Cirelli (2003) proposed the 'synaptic homeostasis hypothesis' postulating that slow-wave activity during sleep has a restorative role in synaptic function. While wakefulness is associated with synaptic potentiation, the slow-wave activity (SWA) of non-REM sleep is associated with active synaptic downscaling that is, depotentiation/depression. This synaptic downscaling occurs proportionally to its potentiation during wakefulness, in order to return to a certain threshold, avoiding synaptic overload and promoting selection. In the following year, Tononi and Cirelli (2014) presented a refined version of their hypothesis as follows: 'By renormalizing synaptic strength, sleep reduces the burden of plasticity on neurons and other cells while restoring neuronal selectivity and the ability to learn, and in doing so enhances signal-to-noise ratios, leading to the consolidation and integration of memories' (Tononi and Cirelli 2014, p.1). For them, this link between the SWA and synaptic plasticity was also seen locally in animal models and humans: a local increase of SWA was recorded and correlated with post-sleep performance improvement after a learning task that involved a particular cortical area. For example, when volunteers without an impairment learned a procedural motor task like a pursuit-rotor task before going to sleep, SWA was increased in the right parietal region the following night and correlated with a better per-formance after sleep (Huber et al. 2004). This was not observed when sleep was prevented. The amount, amplitude and slope of the SWA activity was found to decrease during the course of sleep and thought to be due to the progressive synaptic downscaling resulting from homeostatic regulation and not to circadian time (Riedner et al. 2007).

Considering the ECSWS as a model disease of 'slow-wave sleep pathology', Bölsterli et al., studied the slow-wave slope changes in children with CSWS (Bölsterli et al. 2011, 2014). In their last paper, the authors retrospectively examined the night EEGs of 14 chil-dren with ECSWS and compared the slope of the slow-wave at the location of the highest spike amplitude (called 'focus') of the CSWS with the other sites during the first and last hour of slow sleep. They found on average no change (but a large inter-subject variations is seen in the figures) of the slow-wave slope at the 'focus' between both time points, while there was a decrease of the slope in the other regions, albeit smaller than in controls. The denser the spikes, the lesser was the slow-wave slope decrease. The authors concluded that their findings support their hypothesis that prolonged focal epileptic activity in ECSWS provokes a disturbance of local slow-wave activity, reflecting the loss of physiological synaptic downscaling, and that this could account for the cognitive dysfunctions.

It is noteworthy that the same group recently published a similar analysis in patients with West syndrome (Fattinger et al. 2015) and found again a lesser physiological decrease of SWA during slow sleep. Normalization was obtained after successful treatment, suggest-ing that this phenomenon might be seen in severe epilepsies, but not specifically in the syndrome of ECSWS.

It must, however, be emphasized that the validity of correlations between measures derived from slow waves recorded via scalp electrodes and subtle synaptic changes at the cellular level remains to be better established. Moreover, the synaptic homeostasis hypoth-esis is still a matter of controversy among experts (Frank 2013; Cirelli and Tononi 2015), so that its contribution to explain the impact of epileptic activity on learning and memory remains to be further explored.

In a similar line of thinking, Tassinari et al. (2009) propose to call the negative effects of CSWS on cognition and learning the 'Penelope syndrome'. In the authors' words, 'Spin-ning during the day, spiking during the night, in which the diurnal "spinning" (a neuronal network) is erased by the "EEG spiking" during sleep'. This sentence alludes to the myth of Penelope undoing during the night the tapestry she had woven during the day. This sounds an attractive but is in fact an unfortunate metaphor, because the material learned during the day is not 'erased'. Part of it may indeed not be well consolidated, although this is difficult to prove (see below) and may depend on the type of learning and memory involved.

Furthermore, the variable consequences of CSWS on cognition, including loss of skills that were acquired before onset of CSWS and sometimes also their lack or only minor impact, call for other explanations than only forgetting what has been learned during the previous day.

Memory consolidation during sleep: influence of sleep-activated EEG discharges

A disturbance of sleep organization, quality and duration of any cause interferes with cognitive functioning. This can happen in many different epilepsies, especially with nocturnal seizures. However, children with IFEs and sleep-activated interictal discharges who have behaviourally normal sleep and rare seizures, if any, can also suffer from cognitive impairments. This occurs even if the sleep structure on the EEG is preserved. In CSWS, the physiological sleep structure seems only to be 'masked' and not disrupted like in other severe epilepsies, because sleep spindles and other markers of sleep stages 'reappear' as soon as the discharges become less continuous, during the same night. As mentioned previously, the importance of sleep for memory consolidation has been demonstrated in normal adults and is not the same across the sleep cycles (REM vs. slow sleep) and the type of learning. For example, Peigneux et al. (2010) showed that consolidation of data processed via the procedural versus the declarative memory systems occur at different periods of the sleep cycle.

The possible deleterious effect of CSWS on declarative memory consolidation has become a new topic of inquiry. In a pilot study, Urbain et al. (2011) compared the performance of normal children on a declarative consolidation task, consisting in the recall of semantically related pairs of words. In typically developing children, this recall of learned word pairs was increased after a night of sleep but not after a period of daytime wakefulness. This task was given to four children with IFE and sleep-activated IEDs. Two children, respectively, had rolandic epilepsy and occipital epilepsy, and the other two had ECSWS. They had to learn the word pairs in the evening and to recall them the next morning after 11 hours of sleep. The patients were monitored with an EEG during the tasks so that epileptic seizures or bursts of discharges that could induce transient cognitive impairments could be ruled out. The spike wave index during waking and sleep was assessed. The authors were also careful to rule out a vigilance problem as a possible factor interfering with recall (via a psychomotor vigilance task), because the children were inevitably tested at different circadian periods.

The expected overnight improvement with better delayed than immediate recall was found in controls but not in the four patients 'suggesting impairment in sleep-related memory consolidation'. In both children with CSWS (one with 'a developmental language disorder and periods of stagnation, IQ of 77', the other with 'global mental regression, IQ of 66'), consolidation was also reassessed after treatment with steroids. Significantly, one had normal results after cessation of CSWS and the other improved after their partial decrease. The memory consolidation deficit found in the two children with RE and occipital epilepsy can probably not be generalized to all cases of IFE, because both were particularly 'active' with an SWI of 35%–40% and one needed therapy.

The same researchers pursued the issue with the same methodology in 15 children with IFE, adding a non-verbal declarative memory task – 2D object-location (Galer et al. 2015). The authors concluded that 'overnight recall performance was lower in IFE than in controls, $p < 0.05$)'. However, only four patients completed both memory tasks, so that their conclusion remains to be confirmed.

These pilot studies have opened a new avenue to explore how sleep-activated IEDs may interfere with learning and memory in children with IFE (see Verrotti et al. 2014). One can of course wonder how dense IEDs have to be in order to alter memory consolidation. This is a still an unanswered but an important question, especially for the indication of medical therapy.

A next step could be a longitudinal study of memory consolidation in correlation with sleep EEG findings, each child being his own control and comparing different types of memory tasks. However, the methodological precautions and compliance that are required, especially in the more severely affected patients, should be underlined (see Urbain et al. 2011).

In conclusion, CSWS are likely to impair memory consolidation but several questions are left open. One is how do they interfere progressively with learning? Could it be that memory consolidation is prevented as soon as CSWS start with a cumulative effect on acquisition of new knowledge acquisition? How to explain loss of previously acquired skills? Which memory systems are actually involved or spared (short-term and working memory vs. long-term, declarative vs procedural, verbal vs non-verbal) and how does this relate to propagation patterns and possible distant effects of sleep activated IEDs and to affected sleep stages? For instance, two of our patients with major cognitive deterioration and CSWS with frontal involvement had a good memory of songs and were able to imitate attitudes and words of peers while they were unable to learn any new school material (Roulet-Perez et al. 1993). One has also to keep in mind that memory consolidation also takes place during the day with conscious and repeated reinforcement and that executive functions contribute largely to learning via attention, adequate strategies and monitoring.

11

FUNCTIONAL NEUROIMAGING INVESTIGATIONS IN IDIOPATHIC FOCAL EPILEPSIES OF CHILDHOOD WITH COGNITIVE AND BEHAVIOURAL IMPAIRMENT

Xavier De Tiège, Serge Goldman and Patrick Van Bogaert

Introduction

In the ongoing debate about the differential contribution of ictal/interictal epileptic activity and underlying aetiology on cognitive and behavioural functions (Binnie 2003; Aldenkamp and Arends 2004; Brown 2006; Austin and Caplan 2007), focusing on 'cognitive epilepsies', defined here as the spectrum of epileptic syndromes going from atypical rolandic epilepsy (ARE) to epileptic encephalopathy with continuous spikes and waves during sleep (EE with CSWS), is of particular interest to better characterize the pathophysiological role of interictal epileptic discharges (IEDs) in cognitive and behavioural disturbances often associated with epilepsy. Indeed, these epilepsies are characterized by abundant interictal epileptic activity activated during sleep that is thought to play a major role in the cognitive and behavioural deficits observed in the children (Van Bogaert et al. 2006; Veggiotti et al. 1999; Tassinari et al. 2000; De Negri 1997). Furthermore, they are usually not associated with any structural lesion that might influence brain function. Moreover, in most cases, seizures occur infrequently, which facilitates the study of IEDs impact on cognition and behaviour.

In this chapter, we will present how functional neuroimaging techniques have been used to non-invasively address the pathophysiological link between IEDs and the acquired cognitive and behavioural regression typically observed in cognitive epilepsies. Considering the clinical similarities between the different epileptic syndromes encompassed by cognitive epilepsies, most of the functional neuroimaging studies have pooled together patients with different epileptic syndromes that have as a common feature an increase in the frequency, amplitude and diffusion of IEDs occurring during non-REM sleep (Landau-Kleffner syndrome (LKS), ARE and EE with CSWS) in order to derive the common changes in brain function characterizing these epileptic conditions.

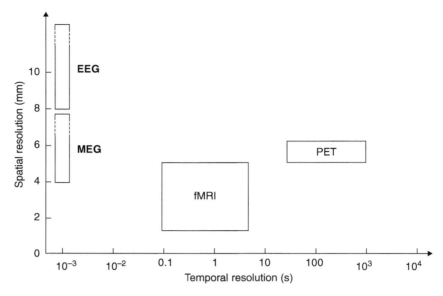

Fig. 11.1. Comparison of the temporal and the spatial resolutions of the non-invasive functional neuroimaging techniques most widely used to investigate in-vivo the human brain function. MEG, magnetoencephalography; fMRI, functional MRI; PET, positron emission tomography.

FUNCTIONAL NEUROIMAGING TECHNIQUES

Figure 11.1 illustrates the respective spatial and temporal resolutions of the different neuroimaging techniques that have been used so far to uncover the pathophysiology of cognitive epilepsies.

Historically, positron emission tomography (PET) using [18F]-fluorodeoxyglucose (FDG) was the first technique to be used (from 1990) for such investigations. The FDG-PET provides information about the regional neuronal glucose consumption via the neurometabolic coupling (Magistretti 2006) with a temporal resolution at the level of several minutes and a spatial resolution of a few millimetres. However, the real temporal resolution of FDG-PET is much lower as transient epileptic activity (for instance, a long-lasting focal seizure) may influence the regional metabolism of glucose for several days (Gaillard et al. 2007; Tepmongkol et al. 2013).

In the context of cognitive epilepsies, FDG-PET studies performed in the awake interictal state are likely to reflect the long-lasting effects on brain function of sustained IEDs that occurred during the preceding hours, including CSWS activity. Therefore one of the main limitations of isolated FDG-PET studies is, therefore, the lack of information on the exact chronology between epileptic activity and altered neuronal metabolism. To circumvent that issue, the combination of EEG with functional magnetic resonance imaging (EEG-fMRI) has been subsequently (after 2005) used to investigate non-invasively the transient hemodynamic changes directly associated with epileptic activity in cognitive epilepsies via the neurovascular coupling (Iadecola and Nedergaard 2007). In other words, the advent of EEG-fMRI allowed investigating the transient effects of IEDs occurring during non-REM sleep on normal brain function. The EEG-fMRI approach takes advantage of the excellent temporal resolution of EEG to identify the temporal dynamics of IEDs and classify their morphology based on amplitude and localisation, and of the very good spatial resolution of fMRI to localise the brain areas involved in the IEDs epileptic network (De Tiège et al. 2011). In other words, the advent of EEG-fMRI allowed investigation of the transient effects of IEDs occurring during non-REM sleep on normal brain function.

Also the use of electrical source imaging (ESI), which localizes on a structural cerebral MRI the neural sources at the origin of the electrical potentials recorded by EEG during fMRI data acquisition has been used in some works to investigate the spatio-temporal dynamics of IEDs to enhance the interpretation of the resulting fMRI maps. ESI is characterized by an exquisite temporal resolution at the level of the millisecond but a spatial resolution of more than 1cm.

Finally, a multimodal approach combining magnetic source imaging (MSI) and FDG-PET was used (after 2010) to investigate the neurophysiological correlate of altered regional cerebral glucose metabolism observed in patients with cognitive epilepsies. Like ESI, MSI localizes on a structural cerebral MRI the electrical sources at the origin of the magnetic fields recorded by magnetoencephalography (MEG) with a temporal resolution at the level of the millisecond and a spatial resolution of a few millimetres (Hämäläinen et al. 1993). The combination of MSI and FDG-PET takes advantage of both methods (neurophysiological signal, excellent temporal and good spatial resolutions for MSI; neurometabolic signal, poor temporal and good spatial resolutions for FDG-PET) to better characterize the neurophysiological mechanisms accounting for the long-lasting metabolic repercussions of the intense epileptic activity observed during sleep.

Long-lasting changes in brain function associated with CSWS activity

Our group initially used FDG-PET in patients with CSWS to assess the long-lasting effects of CSWS activity on brain function at the resting awake state. The rationale was that, given the low temporal resolution of the PET technique, there would be little influence of episodic

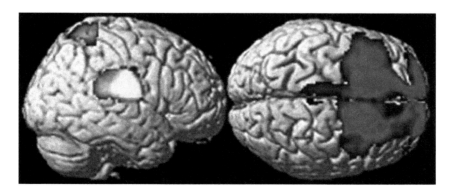

Fig. 11.2. FDG-PET scan: Areas of relative increase in the right superior parietal and perisylvian areas (image on the left) and decrease image on the right) in glucose metabolism observed in one patient during the active phase of CSWS.

IEDs occurring during FDG incorporation on regional brain metabolism and that regional metabolic abnormalities observed at the awake state would mainly reflect the neurophysiological consequences of CSWS. This rationale was supported by the FDG-PET study performed by our group in patients with benign childhood epilepsy with centro-temporal spikes (BCECTS), which failed to find any regional metabolic abnormality at the awake state (Van Bogaert et al. 1998). In the acute phase of the CSWS, FDG-PET data acquired in the awake state have demonstrated the existence of focal increases and decreases in glucose consumption in distinct brain areas (De Tiège et al. 2009; Van Bogaert et al. 2012) (Figure 11.2), with indeed no influence of IEDs occurring at the awake state during FDG incorporation on the brain metabolic patterns (De Tiège et al. 2004). These finding suggested that metabolic abnormalities observed at the awake state actually result from the intense epileptic activity (i.e., CSWS) occurring during non-REM sleep.

One pathophysiological model proposed to explain these findings is based on the 'surrounding and remote inhibition theory' (Witte and Bruehl 1999), which suggests the existence of epilepsy-induced inhibition of neurons that surround or are remote from the hypermetabolic epileptic focus but connected with it via cortico-cortical or polysynaptic pathways. This model was initially elaborated to account for the anatomical relationship found between localizations of CSWS focus on EEG, on the one hand, and sites of metabolic changes on FDG-PET on the other (De Tiège et al. 2004). This relationship indeed appeared to be tighter for hypermetabolic compared to hypometabolic areas (De Tiège et al. 2004). The evidence of altered effective connectivity between hyper- and hypo-metabolic areas further suggested that the level of metabolic activity in hypometabolic areas was indeed related to the epilepsy-induced metabolic changes in the hypermetabolic ones (De Tiège et al. 2004; De Tiège et al. 2008). Finally, the complete or almost complete parallel regression of hypermetabolic and hypometabolic abnormalities at recovery from CSWS was considered as an additional clue for a causal relationship between these opposite metabolic changes in remote brain regions and for the major pathophysiological role of CSWS activity on the regional metabolic abnormalities observed at the awake state (De Tiège et al. 2008). On a clinical point of view, these metabolic data suggested that the sustained perturbation of neurophysiological processes through the sleep-wake cycle might account for the cognitive and behavioural regressions observed in the active phase of the epilepsy with CSWS. These data also prompted us to attribute the neurological regression not only to neuronal impairment at the epileptic focus site but also to epilepsy-induced neurophysiological changes in distant connected brain areas (De Tiège et al. 2004; De Tiège et al. 2008).

One of the main limitations of these FDG-PET studies was that they used a control group of young healthy adults for the statistical assessment of the metabolic and the connectivity changes characterizing the active phase of CSWS (De Tiège et al. 2004; De Tiège et al. 2008; De Tiège et al. 2006; De Tiège et al. 2013). This limitation was due to obvious ethical constraints, which precluded FDG-PET data acquisition in healthy children. The comparison of FDG-PET data obtained in children with CSWS with that of an adult control group indeed impeded any assessment in brain areas with physiological age-related metabolic changes such as the thalamus, cingulate or mesial cortical areas (Van Bogaert et al. 1998; De Tiège et al. 2004; De Tiège et al. 2008; De Tiège et al. 2013; Trotta et al. 2016a). Therefore, to fully characterize the pathophysiology of CSWS activity and its associated diurnal cognitive and behavioural regressions, we reanalysed awake FDG-PET data obtained in a large group of children with CSWS by comparing them with a paediatric pseudo-control group composed of children with non-CSWS cryptogenic refractory focal epilepsy (Archambaud et al. 2013). This study disclosed the existence of hypometabolism in key nodes of the default mode network (DMN) during the awake state (Ligot et al. 2014). This result extends previous FDG-PET data that have shown a significant decrease in glucose metabolism in lateral fronto-parietal associative cortices of patients with these epileptic conditions (Maquet et al. 1995; De Tiège et al. 2004; De Tiège et al. 2008). The DMN is a set of brain regions (medial and lateral prefrontal cortex, posterior cingulate cortex, precuneus, temporo-parietal junction and parahippocampal gyrus) characterized by a high level of metabolic activity at rest and a low level of activity during goal-directed or externally focused cognitive tasks (Gusnard and Raichle et al. 2001). Several lines of evidence suggest that DMN suppression during goal-directed tasks is functionally relevant, particularly in terms of cognitive performance (i.e. the more the DMN activity is suppressed, the better the cognitive performance) (Anticevic et al. 2012). DMN suppression possibly reflects adaptive disengagement of 'goal-irrelevant' brain functions (e.g. mind-wandering), which would be required to be properly engaged in goal-directed tasks (Anticevic et al. 2012). Based on current physiological models of DMN (Anticevic et al. 2012; Raichle 2015), it is plausible that the sustained hypoactivity of this network in patients with CSWS could affect cognition, cognitive performance and sensory processes.

Indeed, the sustained hypoactivity of this network in patients with CSWS might alter task-induced DMN activity modulation as well as cross-interactions between DMN and other functional networks (Anticevic et al. 2012) inducing possible impairment in goal-directed tasks. In addition, this FDG-PET study failed to evidence any thalamic metabolic difference at the awake state between CSWS patients and paediatric pseudocontrols, a finding which supports the primary involvement of the cortex in CSWS genesis, and of the thalamus as a node of the epileptic network involved merely in IEDs propagation, which is not specific to epilepsies with CSWS (Ligot et al. 2014; Trotta et al. 2016b). This study also confirmed previous results from our group (association of hyper- and hypo-metabolism, altered connectivity between hyper- and hypo-metabolic regions at the active phase of CSWS) using more appropriate statistical comparative methods (Ligot et al. 2014). Finally, using the multimodal approach combining MSI and awake FDG-PET (De Tiège et al. 2013), we were able to show that (1) the onset of IEDs characterizing CSWS are associated with significant increase in metabolism in the awake state in all patients, (2) IEDs propagation is associated with different metabolic patterns (hypermetabolism, hypometabolism or isometabolism) and (3) most of the hypometabolic areas are not involved in the epileptic network *per se*. These findings brought further experimental support to the remote inhibition hypothesis by clearly demonstrating the anatomical relationship between the sources of CSWS activity and hypermetabolic brain areas, a relationship that remains less clear for hypometabolic regions.

Transient changes in brain function associated CSWS activity

In patients with BCECTS, EEG-fMRI studies have revealed focal IED-related blood oxygen level dependent (BOLD) signal changes (mainly activations) in the sensorimotor cortex,

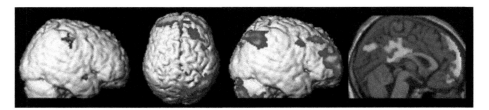

Fig. 11.3. EEG–fMRI: Areas of relative increase (first brain image from the left) and decrease (three last brain images from the left) in blood-oxygen-level dependent (BOLD) signal directly linked with CSWS activity in one patient with this EEG pattern.

well corresponding to IED localization and the typical seizure semiology observed in this type of epilepsy. In patients with atypical forms of rolandic epilepsy, EEG-fMRI showed BOLD signal changes in cortical brain areas concordant with IEDs topography as well as in cortical and subcortical areas distant to the spike topography (Archer et al. 2003; Boor et al. 2003, 2007; Lengler et al. 2007; Masterton et al. 2010; Moeller et al. 2013; Siniatchkin et al. 2010).

In patients with CSWS, an epileptic network that included cortical and subcortical structures was consistently disclosed during CSWS with positive BOLD signal changes in the perisylvian region, insula, cingulate cortex and thalamus, and negative BOLD signal changes in the DMN (Figure 11.3) (De Tiège et al. 2007; Siniatchkin et al. 2010). Moreover, in patients with ARE, EEG-fMRI showed BOLD signal changes in cortical brain areas concordant with IEDs topography as well as in cortical and subcortical areas distant to the spike topography (Moeller et al. 2013). The results suggest that cognitive epilepsies form a continuum of different overlapping EEG-fMRI phenotypes where BCECTS is character-ized by focal BOLD signal changes at the source of IEDs, while ARE and CSWS show not only focal BOLD signal changes at the source of the IEDs but also distant cortical and subcortical BOLD signal changes that might account for the clinical regression associated with those disorders (Moeller et al. 2013).

Discussion

Taken together, the integration of the different functional neuroimaging data presented here highly suggest that CSWS activity is associated with major changes in brain function during sleep that persist during the awake state. These finding might partly explain the paradox associated with CSWS ('Penelope syndrome' Tassinari et al. 2009), that is, IEDs mainly occur during the night and the principal clinical manifestations occur during the day. EEG-fMRI studies indeed demonstrated that CSWS activity is associated with a transient increase in neural activity (as studied by neurovascular coupling) at the source of CSWS and a decrease in activity within the DMN. Moreover, awake FDG-PET studies disclosed that those regional changes in brain function associated with CSWS activity persist in the awake state.

The hallmark of an epileptic focus studied interictally with FDG-PET is typically an area of reduced glucose metabolism attributed to neuronal loss, inhibition or deafferentation (Duncan 1997). The significant increase in glucose metabolism observed in the awake state at the source of CSWS activity is therefore potentially challenging to explain. A local rise in glucose consumption as a sign of high neuronal activity might account for the observed hypermetabolism at the source of CSWS activity. This hypothesis is supported by the demonstration of a focal increase of hypermetabolism in association with intense interictal spiking activity in animal models of epilepsy (Bruehl and Witte 1995; Handforth et al. 1994) and focal non-convulsive status epilepticus in humans (Van Paesschen et al. 2007; Dong et al. 2009). Of note, focal hypermetabolism can be observed when an intense epileptic activity has ceased, since prolonged (i.e. after the disappearance of the epileptic activity) hypermetabolism has been demonstrated at the site of the epileptic focus in an animal model of non-convulsive, self-sustained limbic status epilepticus (VanLandingham and Lothman 1991). Alternatively, a phenomenon of intense 'post-CSWS' inhibition taking place during the awake state might be involved, because a strong inhibition has been associated with a significant increase in metabolism (Bruehl and Witte 1995; Schwartz and Bonhoeffer 2001). Finally, another non-exclusive hypothesis to consider is a delayed high glucose intake necessary to replenish glycogen astrocytes stocks knowing that glycogen is the largest energy store in the brain with a prominent physiological role during periods of high neuronal energy demand (Brown 2004). In that scenario, the effect of CSWS would be dual: bringing down glycogen stocks with a high-energy consumption (as suggested by EEG-fMRI studies) and hindering sleep in its physiological restorative role. The importance of sleep in brain glycogen homeostasis is indeed recognized (Matsui et al. 2012; Kong et al. 2002). Further studies should assess these different pathophysiological hypotheses using magnetic resonance spectroscopy as this technique can be used to determine regional brain levels in glutamate, GABA or glycogen (Novotny et al. 2003; Tesfaye et al. 2011).

FDG-PET and EEG-fMRI studies also demonstrated that CSWS propagation is associated with different regional metabolic patterns: focal hypermetabolism, focal hypometabolism or isometabolism. This finding might be related to the neurophysiological correlate of this propagation, which might vary from one brain area to another. This hypothesis is supported by a previous study performed in an animal model of focal epilepsy that combined autoradiography and single-unit recordings, which suggested that the differential impact of SWDs propagation on regional brain metabolism might be related to the duration of neuronal inhibition; this duration being shorter when associated with hypometabolism and longer when associated with hypermetabolism. Finally both EEG-fMRI and FDG-PET data suggest that the neurophysiological effects of CSWS activity are not restricted to the epileptic network *per se* but spread to connected brain areas via a possible mechanism of remote inhibition. This mechanism is supposed to involve an epilepsy-induced inhibition of neurons that are remote from the epileptic focus and connected with it via cortico-cortical or polysynaptic pathways (Witte and Bruehl 1999). The existence of remote inhibition phenomena has been well documented in different types of animal models of focal epilepsy using various functional cerebral imaging methods such as autoradiography or optical imaging (Witte and Bruehl 1999; Schwartz and Bonhoeffer 2001). Their occurrence in human epilepsy has also been suspected in temporal or extra-temporal lobe epilepsies using FDG-PET, EEG-fMRI or single photon emission computed tomography (Van Paesschen et al. 2007; Blumenfeld et al. 2004; Van Paesschen et al. 2003; Nelissen et al. 2006; Van

Bogaert et al. 2000). Moreover, the regression of distant local hypometabolism demonstrated after surgical resection or disconnection of the epileptic focus are in line with our data obtained at the remission phase of CSWS (De Tiège et al. 2008) and confirms that such inhibition mechanisms do occur in epilepsy (Jokeit et al. 1997; Spanaki et al. 2000). From a clinical point of view, both the sustained perturbation of neurophysiological processes within the epileptic network (i.e., CSWS sources and propagation pathways) and in distant connected brain areas associated with CSWS activity, both during sleep and wakefulness, might account for the cognitive and behavioural regression observed at the active phase of CSWS. This association of local and distant repercussions of CSWS activity probably account for the fact that in some patients, there is no clear anatomical relationship between the pattern of neuropsychological impairment and the location of the source of CSWS activity (De Tiège et al. 2008; Tassinari et al. 2002).

Conclusion

The functional neuroimaging studies performed in patients with cognitive epilepsies have brought important insights into the pathophysiology of the acquired cognitive and behavioural regression observed in those epileptic disorders.

At a more general level, they can also bring better understanding on the pathophysiological mechanisms accounting for epileptic encephalopathy that is, the epileptic activity itself contributes to cognitive and behavioural impairments above and beyond what might be expected from the underlying pathology alone (Berg et al. 2010). This review of the literature also highlights that specific clinical neuroscience issues are better addressed by combining functional neuroimaging modalities characterized by different spatial and temporal resolutions and different neurophysiological bases.

12
DRUG MANAGEMENT OF COGNITIVE IMPAIRMENTS IN LANDAU–KLEFFNER SYNDROME AND OTHER EPILEPSY-APHASIA SPECTRUM SYNDROMES

Antiepileptic therapy

There are a few important considerations that should be remembered when embarking on medical therapy in Landau–Kleffner syndrome (LKS). These also apply to most epilepsy-related cognitive manifestations in epilepsy-aphasia spectrum syndromes (EASs).

First, one is mainly concerned here with the cognitive manifestations of epilepsy rather than seizure control. Seizures may or may not be present and may or may not justify therapy on their own. Of course, in cases with myoclonic or atonic seizures, as seen in cases of atypical benign partial epilepsy (ABPE) or acquired epileptic opercular syndrome (AEOS) with frequent facial/oromotor seizures, the indication to treat is clear. When the cognitive manifestations of epilepsy are likely to be related to the interictal epileptiform discharges (IEDs) during waking and/or sleep, the objective is to try to suppress them with antiepileptic drugs.

The monitoring of the treatment's effectiveness is not the usual assessment of reduction in number or severity of seizures (such as percentage of reduction, change in duration or days without seizures in very severe cases). One is dealing with language, cognitive and behavioural symptoms that are by nature more difficult to assess quantitatively. These may be either severe or not, recently acquired or present for already quite a while or spontaneously improving or aggravating. It is therefore often difficult to appreciate the actual contribution of the epilepsy at the time therapy is started and to assess its effectiveness at follow-up.

Furthermore, a drug that is effective in suppressing focal IEDs or continuous spike-waves during sleep (CSWS) may have behavioural or other side-effects that can obscure beginning language or other cognitive improvement. In these circumstances, therapy is usually considered a failure and is stopped. One must again insist on the peculiar and unfortunate fact that conventional antiepileptic drugs (AEDs) are often inefficient or can even aggravate seizures or the sleep-activated IEDs (Prats et al. 1998). It is likely that drugs such as phenytoin, carbamazepine and lamotrigine provoke this worsening (Battaglia 2001). These drugs have a common mode of action as sodium-channel blockers, and this may be significant regarding the molecular mechanisms involved in bilateral synchrony.

127

Initiation and choice of therapy in LKS and epilepsy with continuous spike-waves during sleep (ECSWS)

Because fully-developed LKS is rare (Kaga 2014) and variable in its presentation and evolution, it is not surprising that no treatment guidelines and protocol based on randomized controlled drug trials have been published yet. However, much has been learned from observational studies showing positive effects of a given AED on cognitive and electroencephalogram (EEG) parameters in single cases, each child being its own control, or in small case series.

Several drugs have been found to control seizures and suppress IEDs in LKS and in rolandic epilepsy with abundant sleep activation. (See also subsequent text about the effect of IED suppression on cognitive and behavioural disturbances in children with rolandic epilepsy.)

Diazepines, especially clobazam (Larrieu 1986; De Negri et al. 1995), sulthiame (Bast et al. 2003; Engler et al. 2003; Fejerman et al. 2012) and less clearly levetiracetam (LEV) (Atkins 2010; Shamdeen et al. 2012; Bjornaes et al. 2013) have shown to be effective in mostly open non-controlled studies.

Veggiotti et al. (2012) reviewed 20 studies on the treatment of ECSWS published since 1986. Most included only a few patients. Eleven were prospective and included cases with lesional and non-lesional ECSW. Diazepines and a combination of valproate (VPA) ethosuximide (ETX) (Liukkonen et al. 2010), LEV, sulthiame and steroids were often effective. Since then, a few additional studies have been published (Fejerman et al. 2012; Bjornaes et al. 2013; Chen et al. 2014). In a small placebo-controlled double-blind cross-over study on sleep-activated IEDs (n=18 children), Bjornaes et al. (2013) reported a statistically significant reduction of the spike index (actually only from a spike index of 56 to 37) after 3 months treatment with LEV. No comment was given on positive cognitive effects, but three patients discontinued the study because of negative cognitive side-effects.

In 25 children with 'idiopathic focal epilepsies associated with encephalopathy related to status epilepticus during sleep', Fejerman et al. (2012) found that the add-on of sulthiame at a mean of dose of 14mg/kg/day (high dose; usual dose in RE 3-10mg/kg/day) improved seizure control (21 were seizure-free, 3 had significant reduction) as well as the EEG in 96% of cases: CSWS disappeared (replaced by centro-temporal spikes in 48%) and the EEG normalized in the others. Only one had persistent CSWS. The authors noted that the effect of sulthiame on CSWS was already visible in less than 3 months and was maintained during the 4-year-follow-up. They also mention significant improvement in IQ and school performance without further details.

Clobazam (CLB) and sulthiame (when available) are currently the first-line drugs, while a combination of VPA and ETX or LEV is another possible choice. The effect of these drugs is sometimes only short-lasting (escape phenomenon), but long-lasting in others, so that a trial is justified. An important issue is how long drugs should be tried (each in turn or in combination), before starting steroids – the most effective, but more side-effects burdened. The duration of a first or second trial with a conventional AED, if not rapidly effective, is difficult to determine in advance but has to be guided by the evolution and severity of the cognitive and behavioural impairments. One advantage is that the often-feared choice of steroids will be easier to accept, after conventional AEDs have failed.

Steriods can be justified as the initial choice in patients with severe deficits and abundant IEDs or CSWS without any hint of remission, after a long-standing or rapidly progressive course. Major suffering for the child and family disruption can also be an indication to start steroids quickly. A family whose child already had months of unsuccessful and/or ill-tolerated AEDs may lose confidence in medicine, and the child may be lost to follow-up, whereas steroids could have changed the disease course.

Finally, one must always remember that, as with other epilepsies, it is sometimes worth to try again a drug that was ineffective or had side-effects when the child was much younger. This may be especially true in EASs in which maturational factors are so important.

Steroid therapy in LKS/EAS

Although there are no published controlled studies on the effectiveness of steroid therapy or adrenocorticosteroid hormone (ACTH) as compared to antiepileptic drugs, positive evidence comes from several sources. In a recent pooled analysis of 575 patients of ECSWS (with and without cerebral lesions), steroids were, in our opinion, more often associated with improvement on cognition or EEG than AEDs, including diazepines that were considered separately (van den Munckhof et al. 2015).

Longitudinal case studies of LKS have consistently reported a positive effect on the EEG and, often with some delay, on the aphasia: This positive response was often seen after all other drugs had failed with a frequent relapse on withdrawal or on dosage reduction in very active cases. The few studies that looked at the effect of different drugs on the CSWS pattern contain cases who responded well to steroids, among them patients of LKS (Buzatu et al. 2009; Vegiotti 2012; Chen et al. 2014). There are several case series of LKS patients that specifically dealt with the use of steroids (Marescaux et al. 1990; Lerman et al. 1991, Tsuru et al. 2000; Sinclair and Snyder 2005; Gallagher et al. 2006) or ACTH (Szabo 2008) showing positive results with few exceptions.

Chen et al. (2014, abstract only in English) administered 'methylprednisolone treatment' for three courses, which included methylprednisolone intravenous infusion for three days, followed by oral prednisone for four days every time. After three courses, prednisone ($1–2$ mg/[kg $\times$ d]) were taken by all patients for 6 months. In 82 children with CSWS, the patients were classified as rolandic epilepsy variants (49 children), ECSWS (27 children) and LKS (6 children). The 'total effective rate' was 83% and 100% in the children with LKS, but there was a high recurrence rate after one year of follow-up (respectively 47%, 59% and 50%). This is to our knowledge the largest group treated successfully with steroids, but the study was retrospective (over 5 years) and not controlled.

The question is now not so much whether steroids are effective in LKS, but to decide if they should be the first-choice treatment, what regimen to use, how long should they be given, how to minimize side-effects and what to do in refractory rare cases or when side-effects are intolerable. Oral prednisone ($1–2$ mg/kg), hydrocortisone (5mg/kg/day for a month followed by slow decrease), short courses of IV methylprednisolone followed by oral prednisone or prednisolone have been found successful (for a review, see Veggiotti et al. 2012), but these various regimen have never been compared. In rare cases, higher than usually effective doses are needed (Gallagher et al. 2006). Whereas steroid therapy is often relatively well tolerated, there are cases in whom the physical side-effects (weight gain, Cushing syndrome and increased appetite) are so disturbing that its pursuit becomes unacceptable, especially when there is no immediate and striking language and behavioural improvement. Like in other chronic childhood diseases requiring prolonged steroid therapy, change in steroid type, administration on alternate days and dose decrease have to be attempted to minimize side-effects. A multi-centric study of children with CSWS undergoing different drug regimens (clobazam versus steroids and continuous oral versus intermittent intravenous) is currently in progress in Amsterdam and better options may become available.

Evaluation of drug therapy, including steroids
Providing therapy is effective on the IEDs, the severity and length of duration of the deficit, the presence of fluctuations before its introduction and the child's age at onset of language loss will determine how fast clinical changes will be seen and the quality of recovery. In many of the early case reports, and even until recently, months or even years had often elapsed before effective therapy was introduced.

The suppression of IEDs and a rapid measurable improvement in language comprehension and expression in correlation with EEG findings will be much easier to document in patients of recent onset and when an effective therapy is rapidly administered. On the other hand, in severe, long-standing cases, there may be doubt on the overall benefit of therapy. Effectiveness in suppressing IEDS is not always clear-cut. One has to compare the amount of focal discharges in the waking and sleep state as well as the percentage of sleep

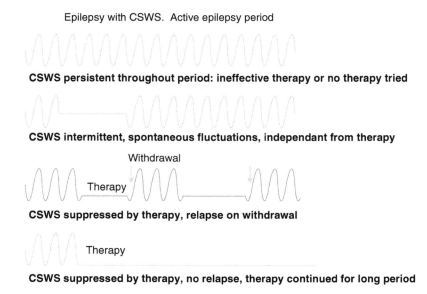

Fig. 12.1. Schematic evolution of continuous spike waves during slow wave sleep (CSWS) with and without drug therapy.

activation and importance of spread over both hemispheres before and after introduction of the drug. Between no effect at all and full normalization lie all possible intermediate changes. Because these parameters can fluctuate spontaneously, the assessment of a positive effect of the drug can be difficult in a regular clinical setting. This is schematized in Figure 12.1.

A clear clinical improvement even with persistent IEDs may be sufficient to pursue with the same drug. When there is no clinical improvement and doubt whether IEDs have started to amend or not, a more thorough EEG evaluation, including a whole-night record may be justified (Deonna et al. 1997). One must keep in mind that the epilepsy's natural activity may be at its peak or is increasing when therapy is initiated. It hence happens that language worsening or other cognitive and behavioural deficits may appear before the drug can have any positive effect, so that there is a risk to discarding it too quickly.

Variability of therapy-induced changes in EEG, language, cognition behaviour and quality of sleep
The overall evaluation of the beneficial (or negative) effect of antiepileptic therapy must take into account all clinical and EEG parameters. These are not simple to evaluate and imply different tools and sources of information. An improvement may be seen in one (or several) domains, while others are not better or even worse. Many intercurrent events during the first weeks of therapy may obscure the possible benefit (infection, lack of sleep and difficult family event).

A striking and frequent observation is the rapid behavioural, attentional and sleep improvement that is often reported by parents before any change in language becomes apparent. These improvements are difficult to document unless specific questionnaires are used prospectively. To our knowledge, this point has not been specifically studied in LKS. By analogy to our patient with lesional ECSWS. who rapidly improved in this respect after hemispherectomy (see Chapter 10), one can postulate a reduction of the bilateral spread of the focal epileptiform discharges or their remote inhibitory consequences on prefrontal cortical areas (De Tiège et al. 2007, 2013; see Chapter 11). Improvement is sometimes so striking that an immediate psychotropic drug effect is suspected. A positive effect on verbal comprehension or expression may be already 'felt' by the child, even if it is not yet obvious to the family and can contribute to the behavioural improvement.

One should be aware that a child who experienced unpleasant auditory sensations or has been deprived of any relevant auditory-verbal information, sometime for months or even years, may have learned to 'ignore' or 'inhibit' auditory input and will not attend or respond rapidly. This can occur even if effective therapy allowed affected language networks to be functional again. Hence, until the child 'rediscovers' that different sounds can have specific meanings, there can be a delay until an obvious or measurable improvement in language takes place (see Chapter 13, David).

Duration of therapy
The clinical follow-up with continuous progress and suppression or marked decrease of the IEDs are the best guide as to decide duration of therapy. As mentioned in Chapter 7, the

evolution of LKS can be very different and unpredictable, so that it is ill advised to give strict guidelines on duration of therapy. There are cases with a single brief period of aphasia, or a few short-lived relapses that rapidly resolved with a short course. A child followed by Christian Korff and Deonna (unpublished) is an example: This 4-year-old child was treated with a short 6-weeks course of oral prednisone and showed very good clinical (aphasia and behavior) and EEG (disappearance of CSWS) response. He had three relapses on drug withdrawal at 5 years 8 months; 5 years 11 months and 6 years 2 months. Each time, he had the same positive response until prednisone could finally be withdrawn after the third course which was given for a longer period (6 months). The initial short course was not proposed because it was considered the best regimen, but because of the brief duration of symptoms prior to diagnosis and therapy, rapid total recovery and the hope that this could be a unique episode. He is now (2016) 15 years old and had no recurrence since the last one at the age of 6 years 2 months.

For patients who have severe, frequent relapses, incomplete recovery, relapses during drug withdrawal and persistent EEG abnormalities, a longer course of therapy (6–12 months or more) is warranted. This is especially important when a hard-won recovery of aphasia and learning opportunities have opened a new life that would be threatened in case of relapse. Many children with LKS actually received steroids for one to several years and tolerated them well. Alternate-day therapy and gradual decrease of dosage allows us to minimize side-effects and to see if the activity of the epilepsy is gradually subsiding.

It is important to know that a drug (especially steroids) that has been effective previously will likely remain so.

A difficult issue is whether persistent IEDs, but at a decreased rate after a satisfactory clinical response, still contribute to residual language impairment and whether this justifies a prolonged therapy to be 'on the safe side'. There are no data to answer this question with certainty. However, one has to take into account that the same IEDs may not have the same negative effects on language networks at a later age. This might explain why sometimes a late recurrence of IEDs is not accompanied by a new language regression.

Other therapies, including surgical therapy

Improvement with intravenous immunoglobulins (Lagae et al. 1998; Mikati et al. 2002; Aarts et al. 2009) and ketogenic diet (Nikanorova et al. 2009) has been reported anecdotally in isolated patients with LKS who had not responded to AEDs or steroids, but we have no personal experience with these alternatives.

Vagus nerve stimulation (VNS) has been proposed in a few patients with LKS and with ECSWS (also lesional case) with mitigated results. In one study based on the retrospective review of a registry maintained by the manufacturer of the device (Park 2003), six patients 'experiencing LKS and intractable seizures' were implanted; three patients had a reduction of seizure frequency of at least 50% within 6 months and four of the children were reported to have 'improved alertness, achievement in work or school' at 6 months follow-up. These are well known but unspecific and not necessarily seizure control–related positive effects of VNS therapy. No information was provided on language except that among other criteria of quality of life, verbal skills and memory seemed to have improved in three patients. There was no further follow-up, which is unfortunate because the effect of VNS therapy is often 'building up' within the first 1–2 years after implantation.

Surgical therapy

Multiple subpial transection (MST) is a surgical technique used in cases of refractory lesional epilepsies in which the epileptogenic focus cannot be resected because it is located in an 'eloquent cortex zone' (Morrell et al. 1989). It is based on the principle that epileptic activity mainly spreads via horizontal fibres, whereas function is presumed to be mainly organized in columns. It is currently performed mainly as a complement to respective surgery (Ntsambi-Eba et al. 2013). It was first introduced in severe cases of LKS refractory to medical therapy by Morrell et al. (1995). Besides this initial publication of 14 cases, 2 subsequent small series (Grote 1999, 14 cases, including 10 of the original Morell's series; and Irwin [2001], 5 cases) were published within the past 15 years showing no morbidity from the procedure and overall positive results. One should again mention here (see Chapter 5) the immediate postoperative effect of MST noted by Irwin (2001) namely that all children, inaccessible and severely disturbed before surgery became calm and interested in communicating. This was a striking, albeit difficult to quantify observation that is unlikely to be reported again. However, the slow and gradual improvement noted post-operatively (months or years) could well be attributed to the natural history and not the procedure, in contrast to the rapid one (days or weeks) that can be seen after hemispherectomy in patients with lesional ECSWS. The better awareness that contralateral independent foci can be present from the start or develop later in the course of LKS also casts doubt on the benefit of the 'silencing' of one single focus. Our impression that MST was of doubtful benefit in LKS was confirmed by a newly published study by a London group with vast experience in epilepsy surgery (Downes et al. 2015). The authors reviewed the files of 14 children with drug-resistant LKS or ECSWS with normal MRI who underwent MST in the temporal lobe between 1992 and 2010. These were compared with 21 similar MST candidates who finally did not undergo the procedure after a similar presurgical work-up for the following reasons: lack of lateralization of epileptic focus in 9, parent's decision in 2, language too good in 3, and observed improvements in 7. Improvement in language was judged significant in only 3 out of 13 patients of the surgical group versus 7 out of 21 of the non-surgical group. Language deterioration was observed in 3 out of 13 of operated patients and in 3 out of 20 of the non-surgical ones, while the rest remained unchanged. The authors summarize their results as follows: 'at long term follow-up (i.e. about 4–8 years later), the surgery and non-surgery group showed no significant changes on any measure.' They did not exclude a 'potential benefit in the surgical group who had a more severe language presentation at baseline' (Downes et al. 2015). Taking into account the limitations of their study, they however concluded there was not sufficient evidence that MST was superior to natural evolution in LKS and non-lesional ECSWS. However, one has to emphasize that the non-surgical group was not fully comparable to the surgical one on several parameters and was likely to have had a better prognosis anyway.

MST in LKS will, nevertheless, remain an important milestone in the understanding of its pathophysiology, thanks to the extensive electrophysiological studies done preoperatively and reviewed in Chapters 2 and 9.

Effects of IED suppression in children with rolandic epilepsy and cognitive and behavioural disturbances

Several studies have attempted to document a positive effect on cognition of IED suppression by AEDS in rolandic epilepsy (see above). A good candidate drug for such studies appears to be sulthiame. This drug was actually shown to be well tolerated and effective on both seizures and IEDs in one of the only controlled studies (Rating et al. 2000; Bast et al. 2003). When available, sulthiame is the drug of choice to treat rolandic epilepsy in Europe while carbamazepine (CBZ) is often avoided because of its potentially aggravating effect and risk of allergy. CBZ is still a first line choice in the United States and the United Kingdom where sulthiame is not registered. Alternatives such as CLB, LEV and VPA can show marked individual differences in tolerability and clinical effects.

With sulthiame, the EEG improvement can be rapidly confirmed within weeks, possibly days (Doose et al. 1988; Gross-Selbeck 1995; Engler et al. 2003). Unfortunately, like with other drugs (typically diazepines), the positive effect is sometimes not long-lasting.

Studies trying to demonstrate a clear-cut drug related effect on cognition, behaviour and learning in rolandic epilepsy are difficult to interpret and have been so far generally inconclusive.

The main encountered difficulties are two-fold: The first is that the cognitive and behavioural status has to be carefully documented before and after therapy with an adequate methodology and with time-correlated EEG recordings. The second is that one is looking for subtle and not necessarily rapid and clinically relevant changes which, when found, may have alternative explanations. In a personal, observational study of 25 children with rolandic epilepsy treated with sulthiame, 8 children showed improvement in neuropsychological tests correlating with EEG findings. No patient was aggravated. However, the timing between the successive tests was too long to attribute it with certainty to a drug effect (Engler et al. 2003).

Wirrell et al. (2008) reported a small study of four children with active rolandic epilepsy treated with sulthiame who had neuropsychological tests before and after therapy. Although the therapy was correlated with a definite reduction of IEDs, there was no cognitive improvement rather a worsening of some skills (reading and mathematics). No negative clinical changes were noticed by the family. These findings were criticized mainly because of the much higher dose of sulthiame than usually given in Europe (Deonna et al. 2010) and were not replicated elsewhere. No deterioration was actually mentioned in several subsequent studies in which sulthiame was used and the effect on EEG and cognition was looked for (Schamdeen 2012; Schneebaum-Sender et al. 2012; Uliel-Sibony et al. 2015).

Large homogeneous cohorts assessed with the same EEG protocol and same neuropsychological tests in the same clinical conditions would of course be ideal but are difficult to organize in multiple centres. While these kinds of studies have been advocated for a long time, none is so far underway. Another option is to focus on small groups of well-defined children with selected ad hoc neuropsychological tests that tap specific skills suspected to be or to become disturbed with time (i.e. visual attention, phonemic discrimination, prosody, reading and memory consolidation during sleep). When carefully chosen in order to avoid test–retest effect, these tests can be frequently repeated and time correlated with EEG recordings to detect treatment-related changes (Bedoin et al. 2011, 2012; Kim-Dufor et al. 2012).

An example of such a study has been published by the Brussels group (Urbain et al. 2011; Galer et al. 2015) in children with rolandic epilepsy and marked sleep activation of IEDs in whom the authors studied memory consolidation during sleep and effect of therapy (see Chapter 10). The methodological difficulties and precautions to use in such studies are important and thoroughly described by the authors.

Practical points and attitude when managing rolandic epilepsy with cognitive–behavioural difficulties

Despite the above-discussed uncertainties, one has to remember a few fundamental data that constitute a firm background to start with when one is considering antiepileptic therapy in a child with rolandic who has cognitive–behavioural difficulties:

(1) There is often no close relationship between severity and frequency of epileptic seizures and cognitive–behavioural impairments. The latter can occur in children who have rare seizures.

(2) Children with rolandic epilepsy and frequent sleep-activated IEDS often (but not always) have cognitive–behavioural impairments (Baglietto et al. 2001; Deonna 2001; Filippini et al. 2013).

(3) Transient negative effects of IEDs can definitely occur in rolandic epilepsy during the waking state (for a recent literature review, see Sánchez–Fernández and Loddenkemper 2015) and during sleep, but the importance of these effects can range from none to significant in an individual case.

These statements have to be weighed against the findings of follow-up studies of cognitive development in children with rolandic epilepsy (Lindgren et al. 2004), which indicate that initially weak performances in some specific cognitive domains can normalize suggesting a sectorial maturational delay rather than a possible temporary effect of epileptic discharges. However, this is not proven since EEG was not done at the time of tests and may have normalized (see Chapter 8).

In practice, patients newly diagnosed with rolandic epilepsy who already have cognitive, behavioural or learning difficulties at presentation, the questions can be as follows:

Do the latter result from

(1) abundant IEDs that started before seizure onset?

(2) a developmental brain disorder that accounts for a specific impairment such as a developmental language disorder, a written language disorder or ADHD (related or unrelated to the aetiology of rolandic epilepsy)?

(3) social or school adaptation difficulties of another cause?

(4) a combination of all the above?

When there are no clear-cut answers to these questions, there is no justification to start AEDs at the first assessment, unless there is an indication for seizure control or a regression. Sometimes, the cognitive and/or behavioural problems are already improving before rolandic epilepsy is diagnosed, an even better reason to adopt a 'wait and see' attitude. This implies that one has to document the current situation, to plan clinical and EEG follow-ups, including school reports, specific academic progress and behaviour and in some cases a first baseline neuropsychological assessment.

In a minority of children, history suggests that the behavioural and/or cognitive changes started shortly before the first seizure. These are very likely to be manifestations of the epilepsy. In others, deterioration arises later with a corresponding increase of sleep-activated IEDS. Optimally this has been documented by serial neuropsychological tests. In both situations and independently of seizure relapse, an AED aiming at suppressing IEDs is justified.

13

SPEECH AND LANGUAGE, EDUCATIONAL AND PSYCHOLOGICAL REMEDIATION

The children with Landau–Kleffner syndrome (LKS), as compared to those with a specific language impairment (developmental language disorder or DLD), or an aphasia secondary to an acquired brain lesion, have often still progressive, fluctuating and sometimes already long-standing language difficulties when the diagnosis is made. It is hard to predict if there will be a rapid improvement with medical therapy. In addition, a worsening due to ineffective drugs or more active phase of the epilepsy cannot be excluded. This not only makes any precise language and cognitive assessment difficult, especially when the child's behaviour is very disturbed, either due to the disease or in reaction to his inability to communicate (see Chapter 5). All these factors can make any systematic rehabilitation plan unrealistic. Often, the child had already received various kinds of support (psychological and speech therapy) before the diagnosis was established. Insisting in making a child with verbal auditory agnosia (VAA) understand verbal instructions or a mute child to repeat words may be counterproductive. One may find for a time a need to focus on psychological support of the child and family. This includes the most important aim at this stage: maintaining communication at all cost using body language, gestures, signs, photographs, pictures, drawings, pictograms and other interactive non-verbal activities. This should be insisted upon with parents who often think one should only stimulate oral language; otherwise, it will be lost forever. Informal interactions will sometime reveal distorted verbal productions that constitute remnants of the child's previous repertoire, sometimes with neologisms, that have a communicative value.

The rehabilitation plan must be highly individual and will depend on the aspect of speech and language one wants to improve at a given phase of the disease course. Brief, targeted re-assessments guided by clinical judgement, parent's and other caregiver's opinions will show if there is improvement or not and if an adjustment is required. Finally, the child's emotional state (mood and desire to communicate) will have a direct impact on his or her compliance with an often-tedious therapy focused on spoken language. In severe cases with total VAA or global aphasia and little or no intelligible speech, learning a manually coded or/and written language is a priority on auditory/verbal rehabilitation (see below).

Textbooks on language disorders in children and their remediation (Nation and Aram, 1984, Bishop 1997; Chevrie-Muller 2007; Mulas 2013) usually include a chapter or a note on LKS without any specific discussion on its management. Sometimes, strategies used in children with severe receptive language deficit are detailed, indicating that the author had personal experience with LKS without this being clearly spelled out (Montfort and Sanchez 2007). Hence, ideas on what and how to do best have to be drawn from different sources, mainly borrowing from principles and techniques used in children with a DLD and adults with aphasia. This includes computer-assisted programmes in which visual-auditory feed-back can be modified and adapted. Individual case studies reporting in details a therapeutic experience, including psychological management followed up over many years can provide inspiring advice that cannot necessarily be generalized. Each new LKS case is a challenge. All existing therapeutic possibilities and techniques are beyond the knowledge of the authors and may require specialized training. Open mindedness and flexibility are the key words, including mixed approaches of verbal-oral and visual-gestural methods at some time points or in certain situations.

A good example of an original ad hoc original approach was that used in a child with severe VAA by Vance (1991, 2001): This 6-year-old boy who was communicating in sign language started to recover some sound and word recognition. The author designed a systematic gradual and increasingly complex auditory-verbal training programme, supported by written language (see later in this chapter), paying particular attention to a motivating content and context (rewards).

Early introduction of written language should be considered. Even though matching letters to sound (grapheme to phoneme) might be difficult and frustrating, like for DLD or dyslexic children, this is unpredictable and sometimes achieved well up to a useful level. It will help the child to discover early on that sounds or objects can have specific representations and stable visual counterparts (whole word and phonemes) (see Chapter 5).

Total communication in children with LKS

Total communication is a philosophy of education that aims at offering hearing impaired or other disabled children all possible aids and means of communication without prejudice towards any of them. A flexible use of those that appear the most useful and efficient, at a given moment, is advocated. They include natural gestures, pantomimes, conventional signs, drawings, pictograms, writing, lip-reading, speech-generating devices and so on. Some of these aids and means (alone or in combination) are presented in methods or programmes in order to be learned and taught in a systematic way. Known examples of these are the picture exchange communication system (PECS), Makaton language programme, cued speech and so on (see below).

The choice of one or more of these alternative means of communication will require a more or less important investment of time and resources and will have to be guided by a careful and realistic analysis of the child's needs and his environment.

Manually coded languages and sign language

In this chapter, one will use the term of 'manually coded languages' to refer to any signed language system, be it sign language (with a capital S, SL), that is the natural sign language of a deaf community, a signed spoken language based on the structure of oral languages or

TABLE 13.1
Manually coded languages

Sign language	Complex visuogestural system used by the deaf community, with its own morphologic (hand configuration, location and movement) and grammatical rules (space, timing and mimics)
Signed spoken languages	Manually coded spoken languages using the signs (lexicon) of sign language but with the word order (syntax) of the spoken language.
Others manually coded systems	
Makaton language programme	Based on BSL but integrating speech, body language and graphic symbols (sign language + symbols);
Paget–Gorman signed speech	Based on English grammar using a set of conventional signs and hand postures together with speech
Cued speech	Aid to phonemic discrimination, using hand shapes and placements in combination with mouth movements of speech in order to discriminate the different phonemes
Dactylology	Manually coded alphabet

another conventional signed system (see Table 13.1). Despite this fundamental and other differences, manually coded languages have in common that the articulators are the hands and that the perceptual system required for comprehension is vision.

One must distinguish sign language used by the deaf community in a given region or country and the different manually coded systems with the same grammatical structure as oral language but using the same signs as sign language, like 'signed French' or 'signed English' or the Paget–Gorman Signed Speech system using a set of standardized signs of its own.

Sign language has its own linguistic structure at phonological, morphological and syntactic levels, derived from different components such as handshapes, hand orientation, location and movements. Sign language conveys meaning by the use of space, hands and the signer's face and body (Poizner et al. 1987; Boyes Braem, 1992; see Table 13.1). Established sign languages such as British, French or American sign language (which was based on the French sign language, Lane 1993) have a richness comparable to oral languages and allow a rapidity and quality of communication that are in no way comparable to simplified sign systems or those based on spoken language.

Sign language and the brain

Whether as speech, sign, text or Braille, the essence of human language is its unbounded combinatory potential (Poeppel et al. 2012)

A first point to remember is that the human brain can learn sign language as early and easily as an oral language. Sign language like any oral language can also be learned as a second language at all age with the same variability in the ease of acquisition and increasing difficulties with advancing age.

As stated by Poppel et al. (2012),

> Research over the past 35 years has identified striking parallels between signed and spoken languages, including a level of form-based ("phonological") structure, left-hemisphere lateralization for many language processing sub-routines, and similar neural substrates, e.g., a frontemporal neural circuit for language production and comprehension. These similarities provide strong basis for comparison and serve to highlight universal properties of language. In addition, differences between signed and spoken languages can be exploited to discover how specific vocal-aural or visuomanual properties impact on the neurocognitive underpinnings of language. For example, the visuomanual modality allows for iconic expression of a wide range of basic conceptual structure, such as human actions, movements, locations and shapes (p. 14128).

Data obtained with congenitally deaf signers who sustained focal brain damage have shown the same left-sided hemispheric dominance for sign language. More recently, functional imaging studies comparing hearing monolinguals, deaf signers and bilingual hearing children of deaf adults in different experimental conditions have shown almost identical patterns of activation, with a consistently left-dominant activations in the frontal and temporo-parietal regions. Sakai concluded that 'these results demonstrate amodal commonality in the functional dominance of the left cortical regions for comprehension of sentences, as well as the essential role of the left F3t/F30 in processing linguistic information from both signed and spoken sentences' (Sakai et al. 2005). Comparisons between comprehension of sign language and spoken language have however shown differences mainly related to sensorimotor processing: by contrast with speech that mainly activates the superior temporal cortices involved in auditory processing, sign language activates movement processing regions in the posterior-middle temporal gyri. There is also evidence for a greater contribution of the left parietal region to sign language than to spoken language processing, probably related to the decoding and production of handshapes and movements (sign language 'phonology') (see MacSweeney et al. 2008). The observation of bilingual patients (spoken and sign language) who can lose one language and not the other also suggest that separate specialized pathways or modules contribute to the processing of auditory versus visual forms of language (Marshall 1986, Marshall et al. 2005). An exceptional clinical case of a right handed deaf Japanese adult with sign language 'aphasia' (also involving sign language production and written language) after a left occipital stroke suggests that visual cortex may also play a role at a higher than sensory level of sign language processing (Saito et al. 2007).

Regarding the processing of signs versus non-linguistic gestures of communication (like pantomime), the involved neural systems were shown neither to be identical nor completely independent (MacSweeney et al. 2008).

Sign language in LKS

Children with severe VAA (and sometimes also auditory agnosia) due to LKS are in a similar situation as the profoundly deaf. All large institutions for deaf children certainly always had one or several such children (Worster-Drought 1971; Cooper and Ferry 1978;

Ripley and Lea 1984). Until the eighties, most schools for the deaf had an oralistic approach and the use of sign language was forbidden (Lane 1993). This influenced the education of children with LKS until the gradual revival of sign language in schools for the deaf and as a language and a culture of its own (Lane 1993).

With the recognition that children with LKS and VAA have a deficit 'restricted' to the decoding of speech sounds with spared visuospatial functions, the use of a visually mediated language including sign language became largely advocated (Rapin et al. 1977). The tragic isolation of children who had not recovered and had no substitutive language was emphasized (Deonna et al. 1989).

However, there was no systematic study of the use of sign language in patients with VAA until much later and doubt always lingered that it could delay the recovery of oral language. The type of manually coded language that one will choose to use in a given child with LKS will depend on many factors, first of all on what the child's natural community (parents, school) is willing or able to learn and teach. There is probably no particular difficulty for children with LKS with VAA to learn and use any of them. Sign language or another manually coded language can be simultaneously or successively mastered (see Chapter 14). Most children with LKS who were formally offered a manually coded language at school used a combination of sign language and a signed spoken language, sometimes together or in succession, depending on their interlocutor. In some schools for the deaf, hearing teachers use signs while simultaneously speaking aloud in order to encourage oral understanding and lip-reading, while deaf teachers use formal sign language. This has rarely been detailed in the papers dealing with non-verbal communication in LKS.

Figure 13.1 is a schematic representation of the different language modalities feeding into the lexical-semantic system and their output (preferential or exclusive) in a child with LKS and severe verbal auditory agnosia using sign language (heavy arrows). This figure was drawn by M Vance and one of the authors (ER-P) after the original published report on Christofer by Vance (1991) and during its implementation with our child David (see below). Auditory (spoken word), visual (formal signs of sign language, written word, lip-reading) and kinesthetic (proprioceptive feedback of articulated words in speaking or reading, aloud or silent) may reinforce each other at some point in the evolution (this is symbolized by the '?' in the Fig 13.1), but any of these routes leading to the lexical-semantic system may be temporarily or permanently disrupted or become extremely efficient in a given case. For instance, one child with LKS will depend very much on lip-reading (not shown in the figure) for verbal comprehension, whereas it will be of no help in another (cf. below). On the contrary, the route to the semantic-lexical system used in sign language may become remarkably efficient. For example, David (see Chapter 14) told us about his 20-year birthday party where he invited several of his former deaf school friends (he had no verbal language understanding and production from 3 to 10 years, was a fluent signer and recovered later oral language quite well): 'I am disturbed when there is noise in the background or if several people speak at the same time, but I understand everything if they sign in all corners all at once'. This is a remarkable testimony of how efficient his visuospatial language system had become, as compared to his recovered but not normal auditory–verbal modality.

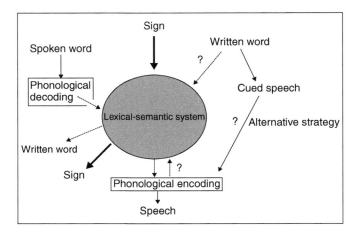

Fig. 13.1. Sign language in LKS. One of the several modalities that can feed into the lexical sematic system.

Literature studies on sign language in LKS

One can summarize the observations published in the past 50 years about communication and the use of sign language in patients with LKS as follows:

'Historical' severe cases of patients with no or minimal oral language recovery, in whom the disorder had not been diagnosed, were denied the possibility of using sign language or their families refused it. They illustrate how LKS can end up in tragic and sometimes permanent isolation (see case histories in Chapter 14).

Children with late implemented sign language (late childhood or adolescence) but in whom it nevertheless brought radical social and familial life changes (Sieratzki et al. 2001). Their competence in sign language was naturally much less than with early exposure like with late second-language acquisition.

Children who used sign language early and successfully for years and who later recovered a fairly good verbal language. They are the best testimony that sign language did not prevent this recovery. Crucially, it allowed them to be educated and to acquire academic knowledge in a mode that was easy and natural to them, like congenitally deaf peers. Their unaffected amodal semantic system was 'fed' and maintained active by the visual input of language.

Children with a relatively short period of VAA, but whose parents chose to engage in learning sign language because they felt that natural and simple gestures were insufficient to exchange ideas and feelings during possibly months or years. The rapidity of learning signs, the positive changes in behaviour and the parent's enthusiasm are remarkable features of these testimonies (see case histories below).

The difficulty in providing quantifiable data about sign language performances has certainly prevented important experiences being published in scientific journals. The rare detailed studies came from neuropsychologists primarily focusing on theoretical issues such as the comparison of children with acquired VAA with deaf children or language development in the case of auditory deprivation during a critical developmental period. Bishop (1982) compared oral language comprehension of nine older children with LKS (10–14 years) with that of profoundly deaf children and found the same deficit that she concluded to be a 'secondary consequence of their reliance on the visual modality to learn grammar'. Eight out of nine used some form of manually coded language, but only two used British sign language (BSL). It was not specified how much they had recovered at the time of testing and how efficient they were in their use of signs.

Baynes et al. (1998) studied a 27-year-old woman with sequelae of VAA that had occurred at the age of 4 years. They reported detailed data on spoken, written and signed English, the latter being her preferred mode of communication (rather than American sign language, ASL). They found preserved sign 'phonology' (i.e. use of hand shapes) despite marked impairment of spoken language phonology. Morphosyntactic analysis of ASL showed problems 'with inflectional agreements, strict sub-categorization, and a poverty of embedded structures'. These were thought to be the result of poor exposure to ASL.

Sieratzki et al. (2001) published a case study of a 26-year-old man who developed VAA at the age of 5 years and recovered minimal useful oral speech .From the age of 7–12 years he was taught in spoken English accompanied by the Paget–Gorman Signed Speech system in a school for speech and language impaired children. Only at the age of 13 did he enter a school for the deaf where he learned BSL, which became his most effective means of communication. He had good vocabulary, but serious grammatical limitations. His mother has also learned BSL and has subsequently become a professional BSL interpreter!

It is noteworthy that despite training, the child developed no lip-reading abilities. This illustrates the fact these skills can be very variable in LKS and sometimes be lost. This is not surprising if one refers to the fact that lip-reading is processed via the perisylvian cortex involved in phonological processing and articulatory planning that can both be affected in LKS (Paulesu et al. 2003).

In 2001, we published a detailed study of sign language competence in a 13-year-old boy with severe early VAA educated in a school for deaf children from the age of 6. He later recovered good oral language (Roulet-Perez et al. 2001; see case report of David, below). He was found to be as proficient in sign language as a same age congenitally deaf peer of hearing parents who had a similar exposure to sign language. Unlike this boy, many children with LKS who learned to sign do not match the level of congenitally deaf peers and lag several years behind them: this is not surprising since sign language learning is often proposed late and familial, social and educational conditions are often not optimal. Another explanation can also be that the child's epileptic dysfunction extends beyond the auditory cortices and affects the cerebral circuits underpinning sign language learning. Our patient, however, clearly showed that (1) sign language can be successfully mastered by a child with VAA and good intelligence, (2) there was no evidence of sign language 'aphasia', (3) sign language learning does not interfere with oral language recovery, (4) it promotes academic knowledge and success and (5) it can also contribute to the remediation of spoken language (see David above).

In November 2007, at the International Symposium entitled "Fifty Years of Landau–Kleffner syndrome", we presented a review on sign language in LKS and since then, no new research was published on this topic (Deonna et al. 2009). Our article was quoted in several reviews on LKS and sign language was simply mentioned as an option in the management of severe cases of LKS. However, we still do not know in how many cases sign language or another manually coded language is proposed and which of these is most successful. It is also possible that some children are using a manually coded language for too short a period to allow proficiency and benefit to be recorded if they rapidly recover thanks to early diagnosis and therapy.

At the Landau–Kleffner symposium (2007) mentioned, above two of our patients who had profound and prolonged VAA (David and 'Claude' see case reports below) but became fluent signers and later recovered oral language were shown with their families in a film (Roulet 2007). This film was an extract from a documentary produced by the TV company Suisse Romande titled Sign Language at the Service of Others, a weekly programme in sign language for the deaf community (http:www.tsr.ch Emisssion: Signes 12.2.2006).

After the programme was aired we subsequently received two interesting feedback One family from Barcelona realized how limited communication had become with their 6-year-old daughter with severe VAA. After seeing this TV programme, they discovered the world of the deaf by reading Oliver Sacks's book entitled *Seeing Voices*. They embarked on sign language on their own, against professional advice.

The mother said:

We did not learn sign language grammar, but only some words (we worked on up to 200). We learned it thanks to some books and videos from a Deaf Catalan Society (Catalan sign language Illustrated) and saw rapidly a remarkable change. I think it's a shame that so many doctors and speech therapists still devaluate and even ban the use of sign language. It shows a very poor understanding of the child's condition and of the deaf community.

The use of signs was necessary for only a few months, because the child recovered quickly, but the parents remember it as a rewarding experience.

Another child 'Lucien' came to our attention through a speech therapist who was following a boy with profound aphasia and without comprehension. He was found to have LKS, the diagnosis of which was delayed because of a normal first electroencephalogram (EEG) (see Van Bogaert et al. 2013 case 1; and the case report on Lucien below). Encouraged by this same TV programme, sign language was introduced and the child was put in a school for deaf children where he learned sign language with great success and gradually recovered spoken language. He was later transferred to a school for language-impaired children.

Although there is no control study comparing the long-term verbal language or general outcome of children with severe LKS who learned a manually coded language early on, versus those who did not, there are several solid clinical observations and scientific arguments which strongly argue in favour of its use. One can also wonder whether sign language can be lost in case of a severe relapse. We have read this mentioned *en passant* in one or two case reports, but this was poorly documented.

Regarding sign language organization in the brain, by analogy with deaf signers, we are not aware of functional MRI studies during signing tasks of children with LKS who became fluent signers.

PRACTICAL ISSUES

The idea that children with VAA, who once had a normal oral language and are not peripherally deaf, should rapidly learn a manually coded language is understandably not easy to accept. It requires time and much engagement of family, professionals and school. Sign language conveys also prejudices and to feel associated with the deaf community is also sometimes strongly rejected. The unfounded fear that sign language will prevent oral language recovery has also to be addressed.

As previously discussed, when sounds have become not only meaningless but unpleasant, 'like a scrambled radio', as a child told us, he/she may avert oral language, become aggressive and resentful at all attempted oral demands or requests from him/her to speak. He can also become inattentive to sounds and if the problem has lasted for some time, he may 'forget' or 'lose' the idea that speech sounds can have meaning. As non-verbal skills are usually preserved, these are all reasons to introduce and encourage any visual forms of language (pictures, symbols and written words), especially a manually coded language.

It is obviously not possible to state at which degree of severity of VAA or global aphasia, at what age, and after what duration of persistent symptoms should a manually coded language be introduced. Only individual-based decisions can be made. One should insist that the use of a visual language does not preclude parallel (or in the near future) work on the auditory channel, providing that the child is compliant enough. Brief assessments of the child's ability to recognize words or more complex information presented purely auditorily is an index of improvement, improvement that the parents may notice in daily life. However, one must be aware that comprehension can be overestimated, when the child uses contextual clues and not language decoding, like children with severe DLD.

In not too severe, fluctuating or recent onset cases, it seems too big an investment to undertake training in sign language since recovery is likely within a reasonable delay. Dogmatism is here unwarranted.

We have seen variable responses of parents to the suggestions of introducing sign language: from immediate and definitive rejection to initial reluctance with progressive acceptance and enthusiasm and natural understanding and willingness to do whatever could help communication. One mother, in the days following the diagnosis in her 6-year-old child with recent onset (3 months) VAA in whom an AED had just been started wrote in her diary: 'August 4th; while putting him to bed, I speak to him about sign language, I have the impression that he would like it, only the fact that this would be far from home worries him'. In this child, language comprehension returned quickly under prednisone and he never had a recurrence thereafter.

Some families and therapists may consider sign language learning a positive adventure and others an intolerable burden. The overenthusiastic advocacy of a choice that is unrealistic in the child's environment and a potential source of guilt if it cannot be implemented should be avoided.

The child's spontaneous use of gestures and wishes to communicate are a hopeful starting point. The awareness of some parents of the loss of fundamental exchanges beyond the 'here and now' can be a strong motivation.

Besides cultural and environmental factors, there are probably innate differences in a child's ability to use a manual language, as one can see in children with severe DLD who, despite similar intelligence and motor abilities use a lot or no gestures at all, an observation that has been little studied.

The frequently associated behavioural (attention, opposition and withdrawal) disturbances should not be a deterrent for teaching a manually coded language. On the contrary, better communication may improve behaviour.

One may also fear that motor difficulties such as gestural dyspraxia (either developmental or acquired) may interfere with sign language acquisition: this may however not be a major obstacle since movements conveying linguistic information are at least partially processed via different and possibly unaffected routes in the brain (see MacSweeny et al. 2008). A low cognitive level may also be perceived as a hurdle, but in these cases, as with learning disabled children, a simplified manually coded language like proposed in the Makaton programme can be introduced.

Sometimes, there is an opportunity to start with sign language or another manually coded language in regular preschool or primary school under the guidance of a speech therapist and with the help of a motivated teacher. Fortunately, some of the younger generation of speech therapists are keen to learn and teach sign language. A manually coded language is now often part of the therapy in children with severe developmental language disorders (including those with mainly expressive difficulties) and other disabilities involving communication are included in the curriculum of some speech therapy and special education teacher's schools. Integration of the child in a school for the deaf will depend on many circumstances: local availability, parent's philosophy and the capacity and willingness for the school and administration to accept an unusual pupil and to be flexible in designing an individual curriculum.

Some children with LKS have a history of DLD, and in some others, LKS can start very early in development. One knows that children predisposed to develop LKS have an innate or/and early acquired abnormality of brain language organization in the perisylvian area. This can make one fear that these children might have difficulties in learning any language including sign language. If this can explain some cases of failures in sign language learning in LKS, there is now enough evidence that the majority have excellent abilities to learn a manually coded language.

Personal experiences of patients with severe VAA who did or did not benefit from sign language

Each of these case histories and the lessons to be drawn from them are unique. Some patients were part of our original studies (1977 and follow-up 1989) and were seen again either between 2006 and 2007 or later whereas others were seen later at our institution or elsewhere. For these as well as for the other published cases (Van Bogaert et al. 2013) the same case numbers as in our original studies is given for the reader who wants to refer to them.

Case histories

Successful use of sign language or other manually coded language sign language as the main language with later retraining and recovery of spoken language

A pioneer observation was published by Vance (1991) and one of us (TD) personally met with the author, child and parents in 1992.

Christofer: This boy had VAA at 3 years and 6 months. He quickly used natural signs and was first taught the Makaton language programme and later the Paget–Gorman Sign Speech system at the Horniman school in Brighton, England. He also learned BSL as did his parents. Once he was fluent in BSL, a systematic training in the auditory modality was instituted. He first had to learn to pay attention to sounds, then to discriminate common phonemes belonging to words that were chosen to be significant to him. It took a long time for him to understand 8–10 spoken words but after this first step, there was a sudden acceleration of progress ('snowball effect'). Details of his management can be found in Vance (1991, 1997). At 14 years and 7 months, 'he could communicate effectively with spoken language, but continued to show residual symptoms of speech and language difficulty with verbal comprehension still affected'.

This work inspired us in the auditory training of our own patient David.

David: This boy, born in 1983, lost all language from the age of 3 years and 6 months, but the diagnosis of LKS with total auditory agnosia was only made at the age of 5 years and 6 months and antiepileptic treatment was started then (see Fig 13.2). Anticipating what his future might be without an alternative language, he was admitted in a school for the deaf at the age of 6. This was possible thanks to the efforts of several professionals, and the final acceptance of the family despite initially marked reluctance. He spent his entire school years there. He had fully preserved intelligence and no behavioural or social interaction difficulties except when demands were made in spoken language. At the age of 13, a systematic study of the quality of his sign language was undertaken. His performances were compared to that a congenitally deaf child of hearing parents who started to learn sign language at the same age and both boys showed a remarkable and comparable mastery of sign language (Roulet-Perez et al. 2001; see also above in this chapter).

A systematic auditory training was undertaken from the age of 9. The possibility of explaining to David why this approach was needed greatly contributed to his motivation and full collaboration in this arduous work, especially at onset. He finally made a very good recovery of oral language that allowed him access to a secondary education and vocational training as an engine designer in a regular technical school. He also learned a fair amount of English and German and has functional written language. He has kept his proficiency in sign language and active friendships in the deaf community.

The course of David's history can be seen in Figure 13.2 (see Chapter 13).

Lucien (b.2005; case 1 Van Bogaert 2013): Attended school for the deaf for 2 years and returned to a class for children with developmental language disorder.

This boy progressively lost all verbal comprehension and expression within a few weeks at the age of 3 years 6 months. Because the first EEG (including sleep) was normal and because he had had no seizures, the diagnosis of LKS was delayed for over a year (4 years 7 months).

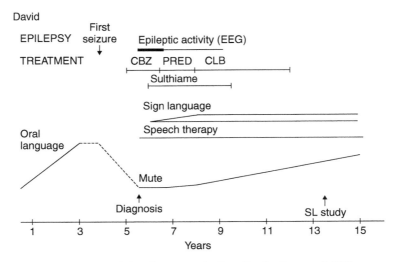

Fig. 13.2. David's prolonged verbal auditory agnosia. From Roulet-Perez et al. 2001.

At the insistence of his speech therapist he was referred to another hospital and at this time he had an EEG typical of LKS with CSWS (see Chapter 9). Therapy with hydrocortisone was started rapidly and his EEG normalized. There was a drastic positive change in his behaviour within 3–4 weeks, whereas language improvement was much more delayed and gradual. At the age 4 years 11 months, communication was still limited to natural gestures, as he hardly understood spoken words, albeit he was able to produce recognizable and context-related monosyllabic utterances. At that time, the decision to introduce a manually coded language was taken and he was put in a school with deaf children. 'He learned signs at an unbelievable speed and did integrate very well with deaf children'.

Soon and with the help of lip-reading, the child began to associate signs and pictures of words with spoken words, which he first could repeat and then progressively use spontaneously. At age 6 years and 8 months, recognition of non-verbal sounds and auditory attention had further improved, yet comprehension of spoken language remained inferior to that of sign language. The child was able to repeat phonemes and simple syllables, but consonants were frequently substituted. Digits and three-syllabic utterances could not be repeated. His vocabulary had improved thanks to the use of sign language. Expressively, he communicated by combining signs, gestures, mimics, intonation and utterances. He often produced a syllabic jargon that limited effective communication. At the same time, spoken language rehabilitation focused on reinforcing and applying words learned visually at school, while syntax was trained using pictograms. At school, the child had started learning to read. As he continued to recover, signs were used much less and at the age of 9 years, he was transferred to a school for children with DLD.

Comment: The long period before diagnosis with severe VAA made it very clear how much and rapidly these three children benefited from sign language. They all recovered spoken language during their stay in a school for deaf children and while they progressed in sign language. This recovery was supported by the signing and they moved without problems from one mode of communication to the other, both at home and at school.

'CLAUDE' (B 1996) TEMPORARY USE OF SIGN LANGUAGE IN THE TOTAL AUDITORY AGNOSIA PHASE
Claude was 4-years-old when he gradually lost all comprehension of language and ability to speak over a 3–6 months period. He soon started to use natural signs, and formal sign language (a combination of French sign language and signed French) was introduced about one year after disease onset. His mother, his 9-year-old sister and the speech therapist learned sign language with enthusiasm. It was also used like a game and the family was happy to share a 'secret language' enabling them to communicate without being understood by others. He was kept in his regular elementary school. He rapidly became proficient in sign language, his sister even more so. Significant verbal recovery occurred with steroid treatment about 6 months after introduction of sign language (see Fig 13.3), with spontaneous decrease of signing. Sign language was his main mode of communication for about 2 years. He gradually fully recovered and has been off all treatment since the age of 10 years with a normal sleep and waking EEG. His family is convinced that sign language was crucial in keeping him a full member of the family, allowing expression of feelings and ability to refer to other topics than 'here and now' (Ref. 1 TV Suisse Romande). At the age of 12, his IQ was in the upper norms (Perceptive Reasoning Index = 107, Verbal Comprehension Index = 112) and his oral language was normal. Formal neuropsychological testing showed normal written language and mathematical skills. The only deficit was a limited verbal short-term memory. Dichotic listening showed a complete extinction in the right ear, like when he was tested previously (see Fig 13.3).

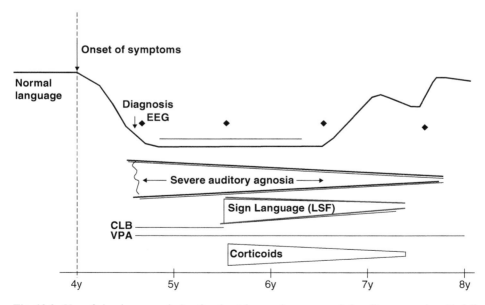

Fig. 13.3. Use of sign language during for about 2 years in severe verbal auditory agnosia with full recovery (Claude described above). LSF, French sign language; CLB, clobazam; VPA, valproic acid.

'Kevin': Early acquired versus congenital VAA with rapid oral language recovery while in kindergarten for the deaf

This boy's history has been reported in the section on early onset VAA (Chapter 5). We focus here on his evolution in a kindergarten for deaf children while he had no verbal comprehension. From the time he entered this kindergarten, where he spent 2 years, he was immediately at ease with the other children and became quieter. He was taught signs by a deaf adult and wondered why he did not have hearing aids like his peers. He realized only at the end of his stay that he was not deaf. His signing was not as precise as the congenitally deaf, but he quickly corrected his mother who was also training in sign language. He progressed well for several months, until oral comprehension followed by production gradually started. However, he continued to sign for a while speaking and did some 'babbling' with the hands which seemed to help him to find a word. At one of his mother's visit to the school, a year after he entered it, he signed with her and did not talk, asked her to sign, took her hand to show the right sign when needed, and as she produced it, he himself then accompanied his sign with speech. Later on, he mostly expressed himself verbally, but used signs when he was not understood or stressed, when there was background noise or if he wanted to give a message to somebody at distance. He knew precisely whom to address in sign or in speech. After these 2 years, he joined a regular school. At 10 years, he followed a normal school and had no residual oral language deficit, but was found to have ADHD. He has only a faint memory from this period in the kindergarten for the deaf and he did not keep friends or contact with the deaf community. For his parents, his stay in this school and sign language learning 'saved him'.

Persistent VAA with good use of two-language systems, no oral language recovery and excellent written language (case 3, Van Bogaert et al. 2013)

'Alice' was born in 1989 with excellent early language development presented with a severe VAA of rapid onset at the age of 2 years and 6 months. The diagnosis of LKS was made 6 months later and she received standard antiepileptic treatment and steroids. She was first trained in Paget–Gorman Signed Speech from 5 to 11 years. She also followed an 8 months course with a deaf person in order to learn Irish sign language (ISL) before entering a school for deaf children, which she attended from 11 to 16 years. She was initially happy there and progressed well in ISL, but felt not as fluent as her profoundly deaf peers. When she communicated with them, she often had to ask them to sign more slowly; her deaf peers did not like 'all that stuff she uses', meaning the grammatical signs she added to ISL coming from the Paget—Gorman Sign Speech. In addition, most of her deaf peers had low literacy skills, and she increasingly thought that their level was too low for her. As she progressed academically, she increasingly felt intellectually understimulated. Around the age of 15, she realized she was recovering some oral understanding and she suffered from the absence of auditory stimulation and of a hearing environment. She hence gradually found that the school was less and less adapted to her. Because of a disagreement with the local school authorities when she and her parents wanted her back in a main stream school and she stayed home for one year. She was finally accepted in a regular school with good support. An ISL interpreter was present in the class and a one hour per week course of ISL was introduced for her classmates. One of them learned sign language remarkably well and became her best friend. Despite her everyday use of ISL, her communication was restricted to her family where everybody was signing even though not always fluently. She was the oldest of six children. She never identified with the deaf community and culture despite years of schooling with the deaf and had too poor oral language to integrate with the speaking community, so that she is between two worlds. The fact that she first used a sign system based on spoken language and was exposed to sign language only late set her apart from them. She was able to acquire normal written language skills. This is rarely if ever seen in patients with LKS who have not fully recovered oral language and represents an unusual instance of 'reading without phonology'. This was unfortunately not studied further (see discussion on written language in Chapter 5). A plan of systematic auditory (re) training she adhered to initially was proposed but could not be implemented.

LATE SIGN LANGUAGE LEARNING IN A WOMAN WITH COMPLETE VAA

'Rita' born in 1965, lost all language comprehension and expression at the age of 3 years and 6 months and has never recovered since (case 4, in Deonna et al. 1989). As a child, hearing aids were tried and she remembers it as a negative experience ('whistling'). She never had contact with the deaf community. The family remembers visiting a school for the deaf with her, but she refused to go and this was never discussed again.

She attended a special school for learning disabled children with whom she had no contact. The diagnosis of LKS was made when she was 10-years-old. A performance IQ of 87 (WISC) was obtained. At the age of 12, she started to learn basic Swiss French sign language with her speech therapist who learned with her. At the age of 20, she joined a sign language training course for hearing people run by a deaf signing teacher. She enjoyed it very much and progressed significantly. A video of a discussion in sign language with her mother was shown at that time to a bilingual sign language teacher who noted that she had some elaborate sentences and that the placing of signs was at a high level for a beginner. He thought that she was an intelligent person who had the capacity to progress in sign language.

Since the age of 20, she was employed as a laundress at our hospital where her senior colleague was a deaf person with whom she communicated in sign language. Otherwise, she never had contact with other deaf people. She married a hearing man, got a driver's licence and was fully independent. She has had a 13-year-old child with whom she spoke in signs. Her knowledge of written language was elementary. She was able to understand simple words and written questions and uses short text messages. In 2007, one of us (TD) happened to see her by chance sitting on a terrace of a café in Lausanne chatting rapidly in signs with a young man. Her mother thought that she was far less proficient in sign language as compared with deaf people.

Permanent VAA of early onset and late sign language learning (11 years)

This girl 'Lina', born in 1986 (case 2, Van Bogaert et al. 2013, see Chapter 9) was hospitalized at the age of 3 years 9 months for absence of language. At the age of 6 months, she was babbling; at the age 18 months, she had a few single words and at the age of 2 years, she had 10 words but no word associations. Understanding was reported as normal at that time. At the age of 2 years 6 months, just after starting kindergarten, she completely lost her ability to speak within a few weeks and was first considered deaf. Brainstem auditory evoked potentials showed normal auditory thresholds. A psychiatrist evoked a diagnosis of psychic trauma.

At examination (3 years 9 months), the child was able to express herself by mimicking and gestures but she could not understand any verbal message nor recognize any familiar noise. The profile was consistent with auditory and VAA. Neurological examination was normal. Non-verbal IQ was 110 at the Leiter International Performance Scale. An EEG was performed during a nap. A stage 2 of sleep was attained, and the EEG was considered as normal in the wake state as well as during sleep. Cerebral MRI was normal. PET scan with FDG showed right temporal hypometabolism at visual inspection of the images. She was discharged with speech therapy. A wake EEG was repeated at the age of 6 years and showed abundant IED (interictal discharges) in the right temporal region with secondary diffusion. A sleep recording performed during a night showed diffuse CSWS. Various anti-epileptic drugs were tried, including a short course of corticosteroids at the age of 8 years (i.e. 4 years after the onset of symptoms). A few tonic-clonic seizures occurred between ages 6 and 7 but did not recur afterwards. At the age of 10, she entered a school for deaf children and learned sign language but she never felt part of the deaf world ('they sign too quickly and among themselves' said the mother) where she stayed for 10 years. At the age of 25, she communicated in signing or using pictograms. She communicated with her mother and sister who learned to sign, but via pictograms with the father who never wanted to learn sign language. She became a kitchen employee in a public institution where she had nobody she can communicate with. She is now able to identify environmental non-verbal sounds but unable to understand spoken language. Her learning abilities remain low and her level in sign language is considered as weak. Surprisingly, she is able to write short messages on her mobile phone, take pictures and use Facebook, despite her poor written skills. An example of her messages in French in exactly the same words is given here 'oui je suis seul fatigues moi journnée chefs' 'non chez mère avec moi je venir maman!, pas tu boulot moi demain je en sais pas oki'. She uses earphones when looking at a movie and probably gets some meaning from certain auditory clues. She is unable to live independently according to the mother, although she would like to.

This story illustrates better than any other the complexity of these situations and the obstacles on the way to implement a visually coded language. Part of the failure of fluent sign language acquisition and low learning skills in general may be explained here not only by late exposure and psychological reasons but also by the consequences of the longstanding epileptic activity that may have affected permanently the whole language and more widespread 'cognitive' networks.

Unsuccessful or no use of sign language or other manually coded language
SEVERE PERMANENT AUDITORY AGNOSIA: NO SIGN LANGUAGE COMMUNICATION DESPITE YEARS OF SCHOOLING WITH THE DEAF

'Christian' born in 1964 (Deonna et al. 1989, case 4) had the onset of LKS at the age of 4. From the age of 5–17 years, he was in two different schools for the deaf and lived with deaf classmates but did not learn any significant sign language. At the age of 42, he lives in a sheltered home with learning disabled persons and communicates almost exclusively with his family with a few simple spoken words he has retained and can understand. His parents were against sign language from the beginning. He never wanted to be with the deaf people and to use and learn signs. He reads a few words (newspapers headlines), and he understands and knows a few elementary signs. This almost complete absence of gestural communication despite his years of living with the deaf is hard to understand. In the seventies, the educational approach was purely oralist and Christian did not identify with the profoundly deaf and did not consider himself part of their world. His deaf peers who were fluent signers may have excluded him, especially because he was not skilled enough or slow in learning. He had no intellectual disability (Wechsler Intelligence Scale for Children Performance IQ of 87 at 11 years) nor was he autistic, but tended to be withdrawn and aggressive as a child. One can wonder if he had specific difficulties to use gestures as a linguistic code, although this was never assessed. He was independent for everyday activities, so we can at least say that he was not apraxic in non-linguistic gestures. Besides this possibility, one can only suppose his tragic outcome was the combined result of parental resistance, ambivalence of the teaching staff who insisted with an oralist approach, and absence of identification and possible rejection by signing deaf peers. He had years of unsuccessful speech therapy. He always kept some rudimentary oral comprehension and expression that probably also gave the false hope of a recovery.

PROFOUND PERMANENT VAA IN A 55-YEAR-OLD MAN WITHOUT EXPOSURE TO SIGN LANGUAGE AND USE OF A MINIMAL 'PRIVATE' SPOKEN LANGUAGE

This man 'John' born in 1952 (case 7, Deonna et al. 1989) lost all verbal comprehension and expression at the age of 7 years and 6 months and has never recovered. The diagnosis of LKS was made retrospectively when he was in his thirties. He was never offered any alternative means of communication. His 80-year-old mother remembers she begged that he be placed in school with deaf children, but he spent his life in an institution for people with intellectual disability and epilepsy In 1992, Peter and Assal (1992) published a study of his verbal productions limited to idiosyncratic onomatopeias and syntagms (syntagms are defined as a set of elements like words or syllables forming a sequential relationship to one another). The full list of these 'private' productions taken from the author's article was shown again to the institution's staff and his mother 15 years later (2007) by TD in his presence. The 'lexical' stock was essentially the same. The man is unable to read and write and his non-verbal IQ in 1992 was 65. He uses a few simple gestures and has no behavioural difficulties. He is autonomous in the sheltered environment where he lives with other disabled persons (none is deaf). TD witnessed his mother explaining him in her own gestural code that she had come that day only to talk to TD and that he should wait another two days to come home for Easter. He seemed to have understood.

ORAL LANGUAGE RECOVERY DESPITE PROLONGED DEPRIVATION OF COMMUNICATION DURING CHILDHOOD (NO IMPLEMENTATION OF A MANUALLY CODED LANGUAGE)

This French girl, 'Mireille' born in 1986, lost all verbal comprehension over a 2-week-period at the age of 3 years 2 months. The diagnosis of VAA was made rapidly, and she was treated with steroids for several years with EEG improvement. Despite this, she remained with severe comprehension difficulties and only limited conversations were possible with her until 9–10 years of age.

A manually coded language was proposed early, but for different reasons was never implemented. She followed a regular school in her village where she had no friends, felt rejected and her parents thought that her disease was not understood. We have followed her regularly with formal language and cognitive assessments from the age of 11–19 years and had contact with her parents, speech therapists and her child psychiatrist. She made a fairly good oral language recovery with intense training. She currently works as a kindergarten assistant and lives independently. Only at the age of 19 did she have enough verbal language and insight in her difficulties to express her wish to know more about her disease. However, the analogy with deafness and the knowledge that some children used sign language successfully was a source of irritation and not a topic to address with her and her parents. They all three remained bitter and angry against the school where M. was so isolated. She never had close friends until recently.

It is difficult to measure in retrospect the degree of isolation, unhappiness and anger of the patient and her family against the school and other professionals and how it would have been different if an efficient mode of communication had been established. It underlines the importance of explaining to the family and the team around the child the nature and the reasons for implementing a manually coded language in order to overcome prejudices and promote communication and interaction with peers.

Lessons from the unique experience of sign language use in LKS and a tribute to the severe cases

It is probable that with earlier recognition of LKS nowadays, more effective medical treatment and awareness of the crucial need to maintain communication by all means, via interdisciplinary work, there will be no more patients with the tragic fate reported in a few of them here. From this perspective, these patients may already be considered part of medical history, but we felt that their life stories should be put on record for the benefit of the younger generations. On a more positive side, there are probably no other examples in medical history comparable to that of the children with severe LKS who lost their ability to communicate orally, learned a completely different and elaborate mode of communication that became their only language for years and later regained their native language. There are several lessons to be drawn from those in whom sign language use was a success.

The first lesson is that sign language learning did not prevent oral language recovery. On the contrary, several persons with LKS and VAA reported here showed that sign language may have even facilitated it, by feeding the 'amodal' semantic system common to all languages, signs or words, thus maintaining language networks 'open' and functionally connected. Sign language was also an asset in explaining to the child who was recovering some oral comprehension why auditory training was important. The child was thus not merely a passive recipient of exercises he could not understand the reason for and could be taught the specific new material, as one would do with a foreign language.

Second, the drastic changes in behaviour, mood, well-being and family relationships that these children showed when exchanges became possible again through a means they could master is a clear confirmation of the role of effective communication in development. From the emotional and cognitive point of view, it confirms how the acquisition of a formal language is fundamental to sharing experiences and discovery of the world. Finally, the reluctance that some parents had towards sign language learning revealed that the prejudices of hearing people against the deaf world and culture were unfortunately still present especially at the time when the older patients lived. Sign language is often not considered a true language but a substitute used by a community of disabled people living on the margins of society. Its richness and culture are not understood by the hearing world. If sign language is not experienced positively by the learner, lack of motivation and pleasure in its use and insufficient practice can lead to poor efficiency and a feeling of inability to master the language. It is difficult, even in the best of circumstances to be accepted, and develop an identity with the deaf community while not being deaf and living in a regular family. This is the issue of biculturalism (Grosjean 1996). It is not surprising that integration into both worlds has rarely been achieved in children with LKS. For those who did not become fluent signers (due to late learning, insufficient exposure, disease-related or other difficulties) and 'felt' or were clearly rejected by their deaf peers and not supported by their family, the challenge was impossible.

The remarkable and sometimes tragic situations described in this book will hopefully inspire those who will have to help these persons. We should not forget that LKS has been for some families and professionals of diverse backgrounds an entry into the world of deafness and to a culture they ignored. Some outstanding patients like David, who is navigating between the two worlds and has drawn from it a great pride and self-esteem, may contribute to reducing the cultural gap between them. LKS can be seen as a bridge. For the few children who had used sign language for a relatively brief period, parents remembered it years later as a positive experience, while their child had forgotten it, as when a child has lived in a foreign country and learned the language only to forget it when he is back in his native country. In unexpected circumstances, a child may 'rediscover' with surprise that sign language had been a part of his life.

In some families, continuous interest in sign language and even further learning of new signs, even when it was of no practical use, has been observed.

From the scientific point of view, the study of severe case of LKS via new technologies such as functional imaging can certainly bring new insights into issues such as successful delayed relearning of a long-time unused oral modality, the occasional occurrence of 'reading without phonology' and the reorganization of brain function with sign language.

14
PERSONAL TESTIMONIES AND UNPUBLISHED CASES

Personal testimonies

MUSIC AND LANDAU–KLEFFNER SYNDROME: A PERSONAL TESTIMONY FROM CHRISTINE (C), AGED 29, WITH COMMENTS BY THIERRY DEONNA (TD)

Christine's story was provided by Marte Årva and Ine Cockerell from the National Centre for Rare Epilepsy-Related Disorders and Grete Bølling from Solberg School, County Administration, National Centre for Epilepsy at Oslo University Hospital in Norway. Christine is a 29 year-old woman married with two young children. She was diagnosed with LKS at the age of 7 years with a typical electroencephalogram (EEG). She had one episode suspected to be seizures, but was not diagnosed with epilepsy. Her language had declined when she was 2 years and 6 months, and for a period of 6 months, she had almost no verbal language (Cockerell et al. 2012). Christine wrote this testimony at our request, which we found amazing. TD introduced some comments in her text to which she responded prompting further comments. Below is the unedited 'conversation' that took place.

> C: *My mom told me that before I got LKS I used to love music. I was dancing and singing as any little princess with a tu-tu and braids. Just before I became 3 years old, it changed.*
>
> TD: This clearly indicates that the disability was acquired, that she had no problems with music including singing and rhythm. Acquired musical disability.
>
> C: *I did not have any early language difficulties either, and learned early to speak. My Mom tells me that my sense of rhythm was intact and that I could follow a melody before I lost everything. This is also a permanent loss for me and an ability that will never return.*
> *A well-known Norwegian nursery song goes like this: Baa baa little lamb. Have you any wool…. My siblings get a kick out of singing it and asking me to repeat it. I cannot hear the difference between when they sing and when I sing. But they definitely do. My youngest daughter (3 years old) says: "It is not like that Mom". Oh, I say: You know, I sing it the Mommy way'.*
> *'I did not like listening to music anymore. I did not dance with my skirt moving in the wind'.*

156

TD: This happened so rapidly, that she started to dislike hearing music. The fact that she stopped dancing may have been loss of sense of rhythm, melody, or both. There may also have been slight motor problems, as is often reported but not given much attention.

C: *I have not had any problems with motor skills. But my sense of rhythm and the ability to repeat a melody has not returned.*

TD: The loss of the pleasure of governing the movement of the skirt while dancing is poignant and beautifully expressed.

C. *I did not like being sung to or being read to. I used to love to be read to. The same books over and over again. I could not get enough.*
The songs we used to sing together, the music I used to listen and dance to, over and over again. Suddenly it disappeared.

TD: Lost paradise of music and dance. The refusal to be sung or read to is probably the reaction to the intolerable loss of meaning and distortion of music and words sounds.

C: *That's right. My parents tell me that they could not take me to stores with music or to restaurants. They could not play music at home or listen to the radio in our car. I was screaming, covering my ears. They had to leave the store, the restaurant or turn off the radio. Then I finally calmed down. They experienced that it seemed like I got physically hurt, and I can say today, more than 20 years later, that was right.*

TD: The physical discomfort of being exposed to all sounds is different from the disturbing background noise in public places that makes it difficult to understand what one wants to listen to specifically (what older people with presbyacousia experience). It may have to do with modification of tone perception frequencies due to partial neuronal dysfunction. I think there are some testimonies in Sacks (2007). 'Musicophilia' of acquired amusia in professional musicians with special insight into that problem.

C: *I think this requires a more complex answer. The auditory processing difficulties make it impossible/hard to separate essential sounds from not essential sound. Since every little sound hits you a 100% the necessity to concentrate is enormous and has a continuously draining effect on one's energy. When you have had enough but have no option to protect oneself from all the surrounding sounds, then it gives you a physical discomfort. It hurts. After a while I became able to deal with the shops, the restaurants, the radio, the family get-togethers and birthday parties.*

TD: Crucial. There was improvement after a peak of disability. Was it tolerance, habituation, or better neural functioning and did it coincide with recovery of oral language understanding? All this is possible, it seems to me.

C: *My mom thinks it was helpful that the language improved and that I got older. I can only speak for today. The extent of my difficulties is the same as it has been in places like that. But l have learned to deal with it and gotten used to it. Public places like restaurants and shops are not the place to neither have important conversations nor give me new information. It is best if I have someone's lips to read.*

TD: I had also wondered in the case of David and Christofer (two boys reported in the book quite similar problems as you) if there was not an unconscious inhibition of all related auditory information that prevented or delayed recovery, because they had lost any interest or even could not conceive that sounds could have meaning until gradually they were made systematically attentive to. This may be pure speculation and both boys had a very prolonged severe auditory agnosia and were fluent signers.

C: But something was changed. I did not entertain at parties anymore, my curiosity was somewhat lost and I was no longer a chatterbox for anyone who showed interest. My endurance was weak and I withdrew from social settings.

TD: Remarkable how insightful you are. Something had changed and that affected the way you were in the world.

C: I do not have a lot of memories from kindergarten. I do remember the frustration, anger and despair. These are the feelings I mostly remember. But I have read the reports from nursery school and it is not a pleasant read. I was not able to interact with other children. They did not understand me, and I did not understand them. Nor did I understand the rules of play nor understand when they suddenly switched into a new game. It was a lot of conflicts. I only remember in short glimpses, but I remember a lot of feelings.
My world changed in primary school, because now I was told to be the strange one. Previously something felt different but not in the same way as when you realise that it was you it is something wrong with. I cannot explain it in a different way. When I get "enough" of music, I get physically hurt. It aches in every tiny cell and all I want is to be in a place with complete silence.
It almost feels like I have overeaten, something I believe everybody has done once or twice. I am so full that I cannot get a single bite down and my body aches.
I get the same feeling with any other sound. It comes to a point when I cannot cope with the noise, and it hurts if I do not get away. I do not distinguish between music and other sounds when it comes to getting "enough" or being overfed to follow the example further.

TD: I have never heard anybody expressing the feelings above in this way and the amazing analogy with excessive overeating. It must mean a very basic overburdening of the auditory system.

C: I was diagnosed with myalgic encephalopathy but the diagnosis was changed into "overload" because of LKS. I welcome any suggestion to normalize the system. Because it still feels like everything is running at full speed.
After some time I started singing again, with all my heart, but the words were not the same as before.

TD: Continued progress, motivation to sing despite double difficulty with melody and word meaning.

C: I only kept concerts at home; it was only at home I was the dancing and singing girl in a tu-tu.

TD: Progress also with rhythm and motor ability?

C: My sense of rhythm and ability to reproduce melodies has not improved. But I sung a lot. It was only my mom and dad that understood what I was singing. My singing became clearer after a while. Most of my family find it amusing to hear me sing. They consider me completely tone deaf.
Music in kindergarten and at school felt terrible for me. The music limited my chance to talk to others, and to understand what was being said around me. I got restless and got told off. At times when my restlessness was a disturbance, the teacher sent me out of the classroom. Then I got the peace and quiet I longed for.

TD: This is the first testimony I have heard of the feeling of isolation from other children due to poor musical ability, that is the important role of music in social development (non-verbal communication among peers, feeling of group belonging, common activities etc.).
In addition, she also alludes to the fact that background music prevented her from understanding verbal messages, and that it must be very frustrating. I wonder how much teachers put music in the background while teaching verbally facts, behaviours etc.

C: I have not looked at it this way before, and cannot say that it is a lack of musical ability. If so a lot of people should feel isolated. Ha ha!
But back to the point: My belief is that when you struggle with the fundamentals, communication, language, speech and understanding. Imagine that you put all of this into a large pot. Then you add a completely new language, the musical language, with all its tones, rhythms, melodies, lyrics and instruments. Then you stir around to get a coherent mass. Then you are asked to find a single ingredient in the mass. This is not possible because it is all mixed together. You cannot separate the different ingredients from each other. This is what really gives a feeling of isolation.
It's wrong to say that I do not get any pleasure from music today, but certain conditions must be met. I take a choice in regards to what I listen to. My choice of genre depends on my state of mind, if I'm tired. There is something about the tones, all the tones that dances in a song. When I'm listening to music I cannot relate to anything else. I prefer to listen to music alone.

TD: Clearly you cannot hear music and do other things at the same time (variable among people anyway). But what music you like, dislike, when etc., would be very interesting to ask, but how. Here musicians could help. Is it a question of speed rhythm, tone, or a combination of these? there are many possibilities.
Here a specific questionnaire on that might be interesting; have you learned solfège or a musical instrument?

C: The music lessons in school were a terrible experience due to tuition combined with music, instruments and a lot of other pupils. Absolutely horrific. I never learned to play the flute and I did not like it whatsoever.
I very rarely perceive the words in a song. I cannot reproduce the melody or rhythm. To the great delight of my family, my family members find this amusing. I do not manage to sing a melody even though I sing it again and again.

TD: This last sentence to me shows the difficulty 'normal people' have in imagining the suffering that can be behind this, otherwise they would not laugh. They probably find it 'cute', or amusing. I keep experiencing this with Miriam my wife, who is severely dyslexic and has to speak French while her mother tongue is Hebrew. Her mistakes in pronouncing some sounds in French are due to her very poor auditory discrimination of the complex French sounds, but people find it 'cute'.

This reminds also of what C. said that people do not understand her problems

C: I often get questions about my accent, where I am from. They ask if both my parents are Norwegian, and so on, I am told that I have a charming accent.
It is more difficult to talk linguistically correct when I am tired. Sometimes I stutter, forget words, forget the pronunciation of a word or put pressure on the wrong syllable etc. When I like a song very much I translate the text, to find out what it is about. Sometimes I get very surprised.

TD: Very interesting. Why are you curious to know the meaning of the words in the song? Because the music provokes you some particular emotions (joy, sadness, etc.?) Or you associate it with a specific memory context with which the music is associated (first love, church service, other devotional act?) i.e. a cognitive component.

C: It is not so strange. Don't you notice the content in a song when you listen to music? Most of the time I do not hear the words, I just enjoy the music.
Let's take an example: My dear husband has a total recall when it comes to songs, the name of the groups and the name of the songs. I do not need to mention who is the best at this but when I identify a song I get a lot of cheers and praise.
The songs I remember best are from the time I went to middle school. When Backstreet Boys, Robbie Williams, Bryan Adams etc. was popular. Since I translated and memorized these songs I am able recognize them. If I do not learn them by heart I am unable to remember and cannot recognize the songs nor tell the name of the song or who sings it.
Sometimes translating a song gives the song a meaning and makes it beautiful. My grandfather died 3 years ago. The grandchildren were to find a song, to him from us, which was to be sung in church by a performer.
When I first heard it, it did not make much sense. But when I got to myself, begun to translate the lyrics, then it gave meaning. And now it means a lot to me. The performer sung the song in a much more melancholic version, it became beautiful. I can conclude that translations give what you hear a meaning. I do not translate every song. The last one was the song to my grandfather.

WRITTEN TESTIMONY ON SIGN LANGUAGE EXPERIENCE BY DAVID, 32 AGE YEARS[1]
Until the age of three, I spoke three languages (French, Italian and the dialect of my home town Bari). After the epileptic seizure, I lost these three beautiful languages and I became deaf. Impossible to hear a sound or music and I was placed

---

[1]Translated from his written French to English by TD. See also the case report in Chapter 13.

in a special school until I entered a school for the deaf at the age of six years. In this school I started to learn sign language which was very advantageous to communicate with my deaf friends, while I still did not hear nor spoke.

At the age of 9 years I started to hear sounds, but I did not know what it was or where they came from. With the speech therapist, I learned the different sounds and learned how to speak. But I had hard times to make sentences and it made me nervous. In the class, when one needed to concentrate on the work given by the professor, I would raise my head to any thing that made a sound to know what kind of noise it was....

Only the speech therapist the teacher and my parents could help to improve my speech. I also learned from my hearing friends, though I was put aside by my hearing friends, because I could not follow in group discussions..... It took time until I could adapt with my hearing friends with whom I was going on well.

While still in the deaf school, I remember I made a test with the hospital to compare my differences with my old good pal Thibaud (TD: congenitally deaf) and was told I passed the tests in sign language (like him) and it made me very happy. This is a thing which gave me strength to progress in sign language....

.... I became fond of music much later around 14–15 years-thanks to a friend I played football with in my village ..... Still today, I work alone in my office with my music, also now to write a book on my history.

ENCOUNTER BETWEEN DAVID AND 'ALICE' A YOUNG LADY WITH SEVERE LKS, ALSO EDUCATED WITH THE DEAF AND THEIR FAMILIES

Meeting with parents and their daughter Alice (see case Alice p. 159) 18 years and David (mentioned above) aged 25 at the time (see case p. 147) and his 'fiancée'. David was educated in a deaf school from 6 to 16 years in Suise Romande, now he is speaking quite well in French and learning German and English whereas Alice has a persistent severe verbal auditory agnosia.

This was one of the most moving encounters in our professional life. We were reluctant to propose it, because there was no certainty that Alice would recover to the point David had and that she will/might benefit from the auditory training program that David had started at a much younger age. David was very cautious when he realized the differences and immediately understood the problem.

It is difficult to give the flavour of this encounter, where immediately David charmed everybody, was funny, interesting, telling simply about himself and his unbelievable life experiences (e.g. LKS and others): severe accident, his trips abroad, his learning German and English (Köln and New York), the encounter with his fiancée (a charming, spontaneous, young Swiss German of Sicilian origin who does not speak Italian, but quite a lot of French that David is teaching her (she learned French at school for 4 years).

The conversation was conducted in French, English, German and sign language. David spoke a lot to A's parents in English. Alice was much more spontaneous than usual, looked relaxed, happy, took photos and a film of the couple and asked David several questions.

The feeling was that of immediate and intense sympathy, a sense of shared experience mutual understanding and a desire to communicate by any means from Alice's family's side. David listened carefully to Alice's history as I related it to him, asked questions (about how well she was in writing, if she used lip reading, etc.) and realized the differences between his trajectory and hers.

David was obviously the hero of the company, eager to share his experiences, successes and opinions on life and he played this role fully, supported by his fiancée (and us!). Of course, his very good level of oral language recovery, his learning of foreign languages and his overall successes (professional, sentimental, intellectual and social) his tremendous energy despite all misfortunes (accident at 16 years where he lost one eye and several fingers) were contagious and created an obvious, immense, irrepressible hope for Alice and her parents that she could achieve the same. They expressed it clearly. Although it was totally uncertain that Alice could achieve the same recovery as David and that this could be source of later disappointments, there were other positive aspects that I saw of this encounter.

First David expressed a pride in his identity as 'bearer', almost 'native' of sign language and in his navigation between the world of the deaf and that of the hearing. It seems to me clear that this has contributed to his self-confidence. He shows continuous interest in sign languages, their commonalities and differences, possibility and limitations of cross-understanding (he told very funnily how he met some deaf Dutch people during his holidays and communicated with them using sign language and discussed with them the differences between his and their sign language).

Second, he insisted spontaneously on the importance of good written language ('c'est la base') and was impressed how good Alice was with it. It was pointed out that David had very little in the way of written language when the systematic auditory training was started at the age of 10–11 years, whereas Alice could read and understand written sentences when I saw her in Dublin at age 6 years. Third, he is learning foreign languages, is interested in this topic despite his still problematic oral decoding skills (and less good written language than Alice) and this was very encouraging to Alice (His life experience in different languages is remarkable and illustrative of the multi-lingual and multicultural situation of Switzerland. He is the son of immigrant Italians to Switzerland (his mother speaks with an Italian accent) and his first language was Italian (Sicilian?) which he has (definitively?) lost and he was raised in the French-speaking part of the country. His fiancée, also daughter of immigrants from Italy (Sicily) was raised in the German-speaking part of Switzerland and her only language is Swiss-German mainly a spoken language and the Hoch-Deutsh (written) is learned in school. She also learned French for 4 years in school, but never used it until she met David. David is learning Hoch-Deutsch, not Swiss-German with a booster 'séjour' in Köln because there were more work opportunities for his profession as a car designer in the Swiss-German part of the country. Remarkably, he 'met' his fiancee on the Internet in part because she was of Sicilian origin (and that was positive) even though he initially rejected the idea of meeting since they did not have a common language (he changed his mind after his linguistic 'séjour' in Köln) and contacted her again and met her in person.

A final anecdote: at the end of the meeting, Alice's mother suggested that David after he gets married should come to spend his honeymoon (I do not remember if she used that expression) in their hotel by the sea. David's first reaction was that it would be cold there, and I was not sure that he understood the proposal. I told him that Alice's mother suggested that they should spend their 'lune de miel' (honeymoon) there. He asked what is 'lune de miel'? (Obviously, he did not know the expression.) I told him that people go some place after getting married, so he said immediately: 'Voyage de miel', probably he knew the literal descriptive expression: voyage de noce. This unintended spontaneous contraction 'voyage de miel' was beautiful. It shows many things. It is difficult enough to learn the literal meaning of things in a second language (i.e. what French was for him; one can say sign language was the first). Metaphors are picked up by real-life experiences mainly, and you can survive without them but lose some of the flavour of conversation. It must be the same in sign language?

Unpublished cases contributed by colleagues

ISOLATED PRODUCTION DEFICIT EVOLVING TO PROLONGED MUTISM (GUNILLA REJNÖ-HABTE SELASSIE AND PAUL UVEBRANDT, GÖTEBORG)

At the age of 6 years and 6 months, this boy with a fully normal oral and written language development had a first seizure with 'biting, salivation and tense face'. His EEG showed multifocal sharp waves increased by sleep with left temporal predominance. During the next few months, his speech became slow, his articulation deteriorated as well as his writing, without any motor impairment in his hand, to the point that his stopped writing at all. The symptoms fluctuated. Speech was formally evaluated at 7 years 4 months, 7 years 6 months, 7 years 11 months and a last follow-up was made at the age of 11 years. At 7 years 8 months years, high dose prednisone was given for 2 weeks with improved speech, but he became mute after withdrawal. From 7 years 9 months, he was mute for 2 months, but recovered gradually at 8 years without change in therapy. First, his handwriting and then his speech recovered completely. At no point did he have any comprehension deficit (including phonemic discrimination) and significant oromotor difficulties. Seizures were frequent initially, but rapidly decreased with a few instances of late recurrence at the age of 9 with transient speech problems. They consisted of hemifacial motor seizure with a brief speech arrest. This case is an example of acquired fluctuating purely expressive speech impairment in a child with rolandic epilepsy and full recovery. Speech analysis showed a motor-speech programming deficit that involved the articulation of alternating phonemes and syllables as well as reversal of letters in writing. The associated severe oral (to the point of mutism) and written language impairment without any comprehension problems or oromotor dyspraxia has not, to our knowledge, been described within the context of LKS. It does not correspond to an acquired epileptiform opercular syndrome, but rather to an acquired and reversible speech dyspraxia without oromotor apraxia. It is one of the many varieties of discrete acquired specific speech and language epileptic dysfunction in the frame of rolandic epilepsy, hence the usefulness of the concept of EAS.

STEROID-RESPONSIVE RECURRENCE OF PREVIOUSLY TYPICAL LKS (CLINICAL AND EEG) WITH NORMAL EEG AT THE TIME (WAKING AND SLEEP): DR. PETER ULDALL, COPENHAGEN

At the age of 6, this boy had rolandic seizures on awakening with several independent EEG spike foci. He was put on lamotrigine (LTG) with an increase of seizures. He was shifted to sulthiame with seizure remission but 8 months later developed language problems both in comprehension and expression, with a normal non-verbal IQ. At this time a 24 hour-EEG showed CSWS. Clobazam (CLB) led to improvement and 6 months later his language was much improved. Several months later, there was a new regression in language, but two 45 minute-sleep EEGs were normal. A course of 3 months prednisone was nevertheless started with an impressive gradual continuous improvement, but not normalization of language. He was put on CLB and levetiracetam (LEV) continuously. Until the age of 12, he had several relapses related to tapering his AED with and without correlation to abnormal EEG during sleep. His AED was reintroduced and he regained his former language abilities until it was finally tapered at the age of 12. He had a normal IQ with discrete executive language problems. At the age of 14, he is planning to continue at a high school.

Comment: This child started with typical, very active rolandic epilepsy (clinical and EEG) then developed a very fluctuating language impairment with initially CSWS on the EEG. Seizure aggravation with one drug (LTG) and a very good, but transient effects (escape phenomenon) while on sulithiame (SMT) and CLB, as often occurs were observed. Despite the normal EEGs (with sleep) during the second, otherwise similar, language regression, a nevertheless clear response to corticosteroid therapy was seen, suggesting a same cause (epilepsy) for the language problems as in the initial episode. The very fluctuating clinical course from the onset also suggests that the same applied for the variable EEG findings without clear correlation with the clinical course.

PROLONGED ISOLATED EPILEPTIC SPEECH DEFICIT IN A YOUNG GIRL WITH EPILEPSY AND CSWS AND DISSOCIATED CLINICAL-EEG RESPONSE ON ANTIEPILEPTIC DRUGS AND STEROIDS (DR. SARAH VON SPICKAZ AND PROF. ULRICH STEPHANI, KIEL)

'Francoise' had an unremarkable medical personal and family history and her language–speech development was very good before the onset of the epilepsy. A first generalized seizure occurred on her third birthday. An EEG in a local hospital showed multiple generalized spike-wave paroxysms and 3 cycles/sec paroxysms, sometimes correlated with eyelid myoclonias and dropping of the head. Valproate was started and the seizures stopped for several weeks, but re-appeared.

About 2 years and 5 months after the first seizure, Francoise had her first sleep EEG, which showed CSWS and she showed many absences with or without eyelid myoclonias. Ethosuximide (ESM) resulted in minor improvement of the CSWS and focal spike-waves were seen. STM was then added. A few days later the EEG completely normalized and the seizures stopped almost completely. At this time (i.e. on low doses of valproate, ESM and SMT), her speech deteriorated significantly and after few days she could not speak any words but could understand complex instructions. There was no drooling, no swallowing problems and no orofacial myoclonias. She was desperate to speak and tried hard to pronounce some words.

The CSWS reappeared after few weeks, and prednisolone pulses (20 mg/kg/day for 3 days, iv) were given. After two pulses, her speech improved slowly over the following weeks and months, but the EEG did not change and prednisone was stopped after a fourth pulse. Clobazam led to side effects and no other changes. Despite that, there was continuous improvement of her language, she could say new words and used sentences with several words but her pronunciation was still impaired. Six months later, because of persistent EEG activity (CSWS), high-dose dexamethasone, (0.5 mg/kg/day for 14 days), was given and then slowly tapered. The EEG normalized very quickly and until now remains normalized, her speech as well as her overall development improved further. A neuropsychological testing using the Wechsler Preschool and Primary Scale of Intelligence (WPPSI-III) ~2 years after epilepsy onset and 1 year 6 months after losing her active speech revealed normal intelligence (IQ 101). Compared to earlier tests she improved with respect to all tested aspects (global IQ at first testing 88), especially in speech-related tests where she was not testable at the beginning and scored within the upper normal range after recovery. Francoise was 5 years of age at last follow-up.

Her diagnostic work-up included MRI (3T), array-CGH, sequencing of *GRIN2A*, lumbar puncture with glucose and antineuronal antibodies, routine metabolic tests (amino acids, organic acids) all with normal results.

Comment: This girl aged 3 years 4 months had an isolated prolonged reversible severe speech loss as a manifestation of difficult to classify idiopathic epilepsy with mainly generalized, but also some focal features and CSWS. There were no arguments for a verbal apraxia or auditory agnosia. Her behaviour of 'knowing the words she wanted to say but being unable to produce them' suggests a high-level word-speech programming deficit culminating into to mutism. There were no clear-cut correlations between EEG activity (CSWS) and speech onset or recovery, in fact she developed speech problems while CSWS had been suppressed and started to gradually recover while they had recurred. Clinically, methylprednisolone pulse therapy correlated with speech improvement (but not EEG), while a high-dose dexamethasone 6 months later brought CSWS suppression and further language improvement.

Despite the absence of good short-term clinical-EEG correlations, the overall favourable clinical course with prolonged 'epileptic' reversible speech deficit and fluctuating EEG findings puts this very unusual case likely within the EAS.

EARLY ONSET (18 MONTHS) PROLONGED AUDITORY AGNOSIA AND BEHAVIOUR DISORDER, UNSPECIFIC EEG FINDINGS WITH RAPID RECOVERY UNDER CLONAZEPAM AT AGE 3 YEARS 6 MONTHS (MOTHER AND DR. KOTAGAL, MAYO CLINIC)

'Eloise' born on February 7, 2009, is an only child. Mother has 'temporal lobe epilepsy' from childhood and is still on medication but is otherwise healthy with a superior academic record. Eloise's social and cognitive development were normal including early language (several words) and there was no suspicion of deafness, lack of attention to sounds prior to onset of the problem at 12 months. The probably earliest symptom was a disturbance of sleep. She stopped her daily naps. It worsened gradually from then on with fluctuations ('better nights') during the second year of life, Eloise continued to make progress in her development until a major regression in language comprehension and expression with major behavioural problems occurred at 18 months of age. The behavioural-language regression seemed to start rather abruptly, but it is difficult in retrospect to separate what came first, that is, language regression versus the other associated behavioural problems. The observations by an occupational therapist at 19 months, the medical developmental evaluation at 21 months and a specialized speech evaluation at 22 months were all congruent in that Eloise did not understand speech and had essentially no expressive verbal language, in addition to many communicative and other abnormal behaviours. The tentative diagnosis at 21 months was that of pervasive developmental disorder not otherwise specified (PDD-NOS). She was considered by many to be within the autistic spectrum. During the following 1 year and 6 months, she did not worsen, but did not regain language, and her behaviour fluctuated and was worse when she had a particularly bad night. She had an active rehabilitation programme to help her in all domains (communication tools, motor, etc.). At 3 years 6 months, she was put on clonazepam, in an attempt to improve her sleep. This had a remarkable effect, first on speech production with return of a few words within days and several hundred words within the following weeks. Language comprehension improved a bit later with gradual major improvement in her sleep and behaviour, all this to the surprise of everyone. From then on, she has progressed in all fields, her behaviour and communication have normalized and her language is of a high level (written language at superior level). She had, however, several specific and more subtle residual problems typical of children who had acquired verbal auditory agnosia. She has recently had a grand mal seizure, and has had several paroxysmal phenomenon that are presently under investigation. She is also having rare but severe headaches that are suspected of being migraines. The hypothesis of an early variant of Landau–Kleffner syndrome was made by Dr. Kotagal in late 2013, despite the fact that several EEGs, although often abnormal (focal slowing) never showed clear focal epileptic abnormalities or CSWS.

Comment: On the purely clinical level, besides LKS, we are not aware of any other disorder that can account for an acquired isolated auditory agnosia at such a young age, particularly when there is no evidence of focal structural brain pathology and enough follow-up (with exceptionally good recovery) to rule out a new ongoing and unknown disease so far. The remarkable and durable effect of clonazepam has been rarely, but well documented in LKS and is a strong argument for the epileptic origin, despite the absence of epileptic EEG abnormalities recorded so far (only focal slowing). We have observed that this can occur initially (Van Bogaert et al. 2013 see also Chapter 13) The unusually well-documented clinical course showed that, despite some autistic features (absent verbal communication, hypersensitivity to sounds, stereotypes and mood swings), play and an amazing early use of written language for interpersonal communication were present. Data on written communication, various language rehabilitation methods used and personal observations on Eloise's loss and recovery of music/language abilities are available from the authors.

15
SUMMARY AND CONCLUSIONS

The impatient reader often starts with the summary or concluding chapter of a book, when he suspects the topic to be restricted to a too highly specialized field or that it will bring no breakthrough. This book is an attempt to show how a rare condition that gradually came to medical attention in the last half of the twentieth century turned out to be the most severe manifestation of the most common form of 'idiopathic' focal childhood epilepsy, as opposed to the focal epilepsies that are due to identified brain lesions. Landau–Kleffner syndrome (LKS) was a cornerstone in the modern history of childhood epilepsy, because it drew attention to the existence of cognitive and non-paroxysmal manifestations of epilepsy. This puzzling syndrome challenged many epileptologists, because the relationship of the aphasia with clinical seizures and EEG changes appeared very different from what they learned about and recognized as epilepsy.

LKS also illustrates how selective epilepsy-related cognitive deficits can be and how difficult it is to recognize them when they are masked by disturbed behaviour and have a baffling fluctuating course.

Information on affected children has understandably come from professional of different backgrounds and competences, describing children at various stages and severity of the condition, often unrepresentative of the whole spectrum of the disease and usually studied for a short period. While working on this book, we have actually contacted several authors of case reports who unfortunately had no data beyond the intensely studied period, especially on long-term follow-up, an important issue that we have tried to cover but that still needs to be further explored.

With the advent of modern techniques for exploring one or another aspect of brain function, more insight on the pathophysiology of LKS has become available, including the possible role of disturbed sleep function. More experience with antiepileptic drugs (AEDs) has improved management, although LKS remains drug resistant in some cases. As technology improved, case descriptions became more succinct, whereas older studies contained important details that were sometimes, to our surprise, overlooked. The recognition of large families with several members affected by atypical forms of rolandic epilepsy, epilepsy with continuous spike and waves during sleep (ECSWS) or LKS, as well as progress in DNA sequencing techniques, has led to the discovery of potentially important genetic mutations (Turner et al. 2015b). The finding that a same mutated gene – *GRIN2A* – can be associated with different epilepsy syndromes belonging to the epilepsy-aphasia spectrum (EAS) in the same and different families gave 'biological weight' to the existence of a continuum between these syndromes, initially based on clinical and EEG observations. However, one is already moving away from the idea of finding a unique or a limited number of genetic mutations associated with LKS and EAS, as has happened in research on autism spectrum disorders. The combination of developmental speech and language disorder and rolandic epilepsy running in families also raised the question of a common genetic origin. Many genes regulating the development of networks underpinning higher cortical function can potentially be mutated: mutations may affect the function itself or/ and generate abnormal bioelectrical activity that in turn can provoke and amplify the cognitive dysfunction. In practice, in an individual child, the respective contributions of a developmental brain disorder versus an early acquired epileptic dysfunction remains difficult to disentangle.

A plea is made here to maintain our attention focused on the multiple and different facets of cognitive and behavioural disorders in EAS regardless of future progress in early diagnosis, new technologies and epilepsy management. Defining precisely the evolving cognitive and behavioural manifestations of these epilepsies and not only a fixed 'cognitive and behavioural phenotype' remains a key issue not only for an individual child's best management but also for our understanding of the relationship between genes, epilepsy and brain development. What children with LKS have taught us and is expanded in this book can also be applied to understand cognitive and behavioural manifestations arising in other childhood epilepsies and developmental disorders.

The pathophysiology of LKS, ECSWS and cognitive impairments related to focal epilepsies with sleep activated interictal epileptiform discharges (IEDs) has still to be further explored and we are now 'armed' to move forward with better knowledge and tools. It should be stressed that, to be useful, any functional imaging or electrophysiological study (or combination), has to take into account the patient's epilepsy history and data on the ongoing epileptic activity with its precise cognitive and behavioural correlates. This is of utmost importance if one wants to disentangle the specific effects of epilepsy from all other variables that can affect cognition and behaviour. These variables such as age at study, developmental delay prior to epilepsy onset, severity of the epilepsy and AEDs still confound many studies even within a same epilepsy syndrome. For these reasons, studies of children followed longitudinally, each child being his/her own control remain very informative even if the number of participants is small.

For instance, the finding that early isolated thalamic injuries in neonates can later lead to sleep-IEDs and continous spike and waves during sleep represents a unique opportunity to study prospectively their time and dynamics of onset and their impact on cognitive development and learning. Such a study may not only have consequences on preventive management of this particular subset of patients but also provide new information that may apply to children with EAS.

Any pathophysiological model of focal epilepsy with sleep-activated interictal discharges will have to account for important clinical observations such as (1) sustained interictal discharges having more impact than episodic seizures; (2) time discordances between clinical and EEG findings; (3) cognitive regression with variable dynamics; (4) diversity of cognitive deficits but also specific patterns, such as acquired opercular syndrome, verbal auditory agnosia or frontal syndrome; (5) variability of course with and without permanent sequelae; (6) discordance between the importance of the cognitive deficits and the nature and extent of a structural lesion when this is found (e.g. in lesional cases of ECSWS).

Regardless of the underlying pathology, the epileptic activity itself is the most likely culprit, when it comes to explain the acquired cognitive manifestations in EAS. Unlike other neurological diseases, epilepsy can occur at various ages within specific neural networks, influenced by maturational changes. It can propagate locally and more remotely via direct and indirect connections which are already or in the way of being stabilized. It can trigger variables molecular cascades regulating cellular metabolism, inflammation and gene expression and thus modify neuronal life span, function and connectivity. These changes may in turn affect essential cortical regions and sub-cortical 'hubs' and pathways within a single or several cognitive networks and cause either specific or widespread, transient or permanent deficits while remaining invisible to conventional imaging.

Our conviction stems from years of study of these topics, being aware that our judgement could be biased and that all mechanisms involved in epilepsy are not unravelled yet. When reading about a new hypothesis explaining all of a sudden a long-standing and complex scientific mystery, one is reminded of the ironic saying of a too-early deceased colleague and friend, Stuart Green. 'Don't bother me with facts, I have my theory'! This is also valid for us and the reader of this book.

REFERENCES

Aarts JPH, Binnie CD, Smit AM, Wilkins J. Selective cognitive impairment during focal and generalized epileptiform EEG activity. *Brain* 1984; 107:293–308.

Adolphs R. The social brain: neural basis of social knowledge. *Annu. Rev. Psychol.* 2009; 60:693–716.

Aicardi J. Epilepsy in Children The International Review of Child neurology, Ed. Raven Press, 1986; p. 177.

Aicardi J, Chevrie JJ. Atypical benign partial epilepsy of childhood. *Dev. Med. Child. Neurol.* 1982; 24:281–292.

Aldenkamp AP, Arends J. Effects of epileptiform EEG discharges on cognitive function: Is the concept of "transient cognitive impairment" still valid? *Epilepsy Behav.* 2004; 5(Suppl 1):S25–S34.

Allen NM, Conroy J, Deonna T, et al. Atypical benign partial epilepsy of childhood with acquired neurocognitive, lexical semantic, and autistic spectrum disorder. *Epilepsy Behav Case Rep.* 2016; 23(6):42–48.

Amunts K, Lenzen M, Friederici AD, et al. Broca's region: Novel organizational principles and multiple receptor mapping. *PLoS Biol.* 2010 Sep; 8(9).

Anticevic A, Cole MW, Murray JD, Corlett PR, Wang XJ, Krystal JH. The role of default network deactivation in cognition and disease. *Trends Cogn Sci.* 2012; 16:584–592.

Archambaud F, Bouilleret V, Hertz-Pannier L, et al. Optimizing statistical parametric mapping analysis of 18F-FDG PET in children. *EJNMMI Res.* 2013; 3:2.

Archer JS, Briellman RS, Abbott DF, Syngeniotis A, Wellard RM, Jackson GD. Benign epilepsy with centrotemporal spikes: Spike triggered fMRI shows somato-sensory cortex activity. *Epilepsia* 2003; 44:200–204.

Arslan M, Yiş U, Vurucu S, Ince S, Ünay B, Akın R. Acquired epileptiform opercular syndrome: F-18 fluorodeoxyglucose positron emission tomography (FDG-PET) findings and efficacy of levetiracetam therapy. *Epilepsy Behav.* 2012 Sep; 25(1):50–53.

Arts WF, Aarsen FK, Scheltens-de Boer M, Catsman-Berrevoets CE. Landau-Kleffner syndrome and CSWS syndrome: treatment with intravenous immunoglobulins. *Epilepsia* 2009 Aug; 50 (Suppl 7):55–58.

Atkins M, Nikanorova M. A prospective study of levetiracetam efficacy in epileptic syndromes with continuous spikes-waves during slow sleep. *Seizure* 2011 Oct; 20(8):635–639.

Austin JK, Caplan R. Behavioral and psychiatric comorbidities in pediatric epilepsy: Toward an integrative model. *Epilepsia* 2007; 48:1639–1651.

Baglietto MG, Battaglia FM, Nobili L, et al. Neuropsychological disorders related to interictal epileptic discharges during sleep in benign epilepsy of childhood with centrotemporal or rolandic spikes. *Dev. Med. Child Neurol.* 2001; 43:407–412.

Baird G, Robinson RO, Boyd S, Charman T. Sleep electroencephalograms in young children with autism with and without regression. *Dev. Med. Child. Neurol.* 2006 Jul; 48(7):604–608.

Barnby G, Abbott A, Sykes N, et al. Candidate-gene screening and association analysis at the autism-susceptibility locus on chromosome 16p: Evidence of association at GRIN2A and ABAT. *Am. J. Hum. Genet.* 2005 Jun; 76(6):950–966.

Bast T, Volp A, Wolf C, Rating D, Sulthiame Study Group. The influence of sulthiame on EEG in children with benign childhood epilepsy with centrotemporal spikes. *Epilepsia* 2003; 44(2):215–220.

Bates E, Thal D, Janowsky JJ. Early language development and its neural correlates. In: Segalowitz SJ, Rapin I. (eds.) Boller F, Grafman J. (Series eds.) *Handbook of Neuropsychology*, vol. 7 – *Child Neuropsychology*. Elsevier, Amsterdam, 1992.

Battaglia D, Iuvone L, Stefanini MC, et al. Reversible aphasic disorder induced by lamotrigine in atypic benign childhood epilepsy. *Epileptic Disord.* 2001; 3(4):217–222.

Battaglia D, Veggiotti P, Lettori D, et al. Functional hemispherectomy in children with epilepsy and CSWS due to unilateral early brain injury including thalamus: Sudden recovery of CSWS. *Epilepsy Res.* 2009 Dec; 87(2–3):290–298.

Baulac S. mTOR signaling pathway genes in focal epilepsies. *Prog Brain Res.* 2016; 226:61–79.

Baynes K, Kegl JA, Brentari D, Kussmaul C, Poizner H. Chronic auditory agnosia following Landau-Kleffner syndrome: A 23 year outcome study. *Brain Lang.* 1998 Jul; 63(3):381–425.

Beaussart M. Benign epilepsy in children with rolandic (centro-temporal) paroxysmal foci. *Epilepsia* 1972; 13:795–811.

References

Bedoin N, Ciumas C, Lopez C, et al. Disengagement and inhibition of visual-spatial attention are differently impaired in children with rolandic epilepsy and Panayiotopoulos syndrome. *Epilepsy Behav.* 2012 Sep; 25(1):81–91.

Bedoin N, Ferragne E, Lopez C, Herbillon V, De Bellescize J, des Portes V. Atypical hemispheric asymmetries for the processing of phonological features in children with rolandic epilepsy. *Epilepsy Behav.* 2011 May; 21(1):42–51.

Bedoin N, Ferragne E, Marsico E. Hemispheric asymmetries depend on the phonetic feature: A dichotic study of place of articulation and voicing in French stops. *Brain Lang.* 2010 Nov; 115(2):133–140.

Berg AT, Berkovic SF, Brodie MJ, et al. Revised terminology and concepts for organization of seizures and epilepsies: Report of the ILAE Commission on Classification and Terminology, 2005–2009. *Epilepsia* 2010; 51:676–685.

Berroya AG, McIntyre J, Webster R, et al. Speech and language deterioration in benign rolandic epilepsy. *J. Child Neurol.* 2004 Jan; 19(1):53–58.

Besseling RM, Jansen JF, Overvliet GM, et al. Reduced structural connectivity between sensorimotor and language areas in rolandic epilepsy. *PLoS One* 23 Dec 2013; 8(12):e83568.

Billard C, Fluss J, Pinton F. Specific language impairment versus Landau-Kleffner syndrome. *Epilepsia* 2009 Aug; 50(Suppl 7):21–24.

Binnie CD. Behavioral correlates of interictal spikes. *Adv. Neurol.* 1991; 55:113–126.

Binnie CD. Cognitive impairment during epileptiform discharges: Is it ever justifiable to treat the EEG? *Lancet Neurol.* 2003; 2:725–730.

Binnie CD, De Silva M, Hurst A. Rolandic spikes and cognitive function. *Epilepsy Res.* 1992; 6(Suppl):71–73.

Bishop DV. Comprehension of spoken, written and signed sentences in childhood language disorders. *J. Child Psychol. Psychiatry* 1982 Jan; 23(1):1–20.

Bishop DV. Age of onset and outcome in acquired aphasia with convulsive disorder' (Landau-Kleffner syndrome). *Dev Med Child Neurol.* 1985 Dec; 27(6):705–712.

Bishop DVM. *Uncommon Understanding: Development and Disorders of Language Comprehension in Children.* Psychology Press, Hove, UK, 1997.

Bishop DVM. Ten questions about terminology for children with unexplained language problems. *Int. J. Lang. Commun. Disord.* 2014; 49(4):381–397.

Bishop DVM, Rosenblooom L. Classification of childhood language disorders. In W. Yule & M. Rutter (Eds.) *Language develoment and disorders. Clinics in Developmental Medicine(double issue).* MacKeith Press, London, 1987.

Bjørnæs H, Bakke KA, Larsson PG, et al. Subclinical epileptiform activity in children with electrical status epilepticus during sleep: Effects on cognition and behavior before and after treatment with levetiracetam. *Epilepsy Behav.* 2013 Apr; 27(1):40–48.

Blum A, Tremont G, Donahue J, et al. Landau-Kleffner syndrome with lateral temporal focal cortical dysplasia and mesial temporal sclerosis: A 30-year follow-up. *Epilepsy Behav.* 2007 May; 10(3):495–503.

Blumenfeld H, McNally KA, Vanderhill SD, et al. Positive and negative network correlations in temporal lobe epilepsy. *Cereb Cortex* 2004; 14:892–902.

Bölsterli BK, Schmitt B, Bast T, et al. Impaired slow wave sleep downscaling in encephalopathy with status epilepticus during sleep (ESES). *Clin Neurophysiol.* 2011 Sep; 122(9):1779–1787.

Bölsterli Heinzle BK, Fattinger S, Kurth S, et al. Spike wave location and density disturb sleep slow waves in patients with CSWS (continuous spike waves during sleep). *Epilepsia* 2014; 55(4):584–591.

Boel M, Casaer P. Continuous spikes and waves during slow wave sleep: A 30 months follow-up study of neuropsychological recovery and EEG findings. *Neuropediatrics* 1989; 20(3):176–180.

Boor S, Vucurevic G, Pfleiderer C, Stoeter P, Kutschke G, Boor R. EEG-related functional MRI in benign childhood epilepsy with centrotemporal spikes. *Epilepsia* 2003; 44:688–692.

Boor R, Jacobs J, Hinzmann A, et al. Combined spike-related functional MRI and multiple source analysis in the non-invasive spike localization of benign rolandic epilepsy. *Clin Neurophysiol* 2007; 118:901–909.

Boscolo S, Baldas V, Gobbi G, et al. Anti-brain but not celiac disease antibodies in Landau-Kleffner syndrome and related epilepsies. *J. Neuroimmunol.* 2005; 160:228–232.

Boulloche J, Husson A, Le Luyer B, Le Roux P. Dysphagie, troubles de la parole et pointes-ondes centrotemporales. *Arch. Fr. Pediatr.* 1990; 47:115–117.

Boyes BP. *Einführung in die Gebärdensprache und ihre Erforschung.* Verlag Signum, Hamburg, Germany, 1992.

Boyd SG, Rivera-Gaxiola M, Towel AD, Harkness W, Neville BGR. Discrimination of speech sounds in a boy with Landau-Kleffner syndrome: An intraoperative event-related potential study. *Neuropediatrics* 1996; 27(4):211–215.

Brown AM. Brain glycogen re-awakened. *J. Neurochem.* 2004; 89:537–552.

Brown S. Deterioration. *Epilepsia* 2006; 47(Suppl 2):19–23.

Bruehl C, Witte OW. Cellular activity underlying altered brain metabolism during focal epileptic activity. *Ann. Neurol.* 1995; 38:414–420.

Boxerman JL, Hawash K, Bali B, Clarke T, Rogg J, and Pal DK. Is Rolandic epilepsy associated with abnormal findings on cranial MRI? *Epilepsy Res.* 2007 Jul; 75(2–3):180–185.

Bulgheroni S, Franceschetti S, Vago C, et al. Verbal dichotic listening performance and its relationship with EEG features in benign childhood epilepsy with centrotemporal spikes. *Epilepsy Res.* 2008 Mar; 79(1):31–38.

Buzatu M, Bulteau C, Altuzarra C, Dulac O, Van Bogaert P. Corticosteroids as treatment of epileptic syndromes with continuous spike-waves during slow-wave sleep. *Epilepsia* 2009; 50(Suppl 7):68–72.

Canitano R, Zappella M. Autistic epileptiform regression. *Funct. Neurol.* 2006 Apr–Jun; 21(2):97–101.

Cantalupo G, Rubboli G, Tassinari CA. In search of the Rosetta stone for ESES. *Epilepsia* 2013 Apr; 54(4):765–769.

Caraballo RH, Aldao Mdel R, Cachia P. Benign childhood seizure susceptibility syndrome: Three case reports. *Epileptic Disord.* 2011 Jun; 13(2):133–139.

Caraballo RH, Cejas N, Chamorro N, Kaltenmeier MC, Fortini S, Soprano AM. Landau-Kleffner syndrome: A study of 29 patients. *Seizure* 2014 Feb; 23(2):98–104.

Carvill GL, Regan BM, Yendle SC, et al. GRIN2A mutations cause epilepsy-aphasia spectrum disorders. *Nat Genet.* 2013 Sep; 45(9):1073–1076.

Chapman KE, Specchio N, Shinnar S, Holmes GL. Seizing control of epileptic activity can improve outcome. *Epilepsia* 2015 Oct; 56(10):1482–1485.

Chen J, Yang Z, Liu X, et al. Efficacy of methylprednisolone therapy for electrical status epilepticus during sleep in children. *Zhonghua er ke za zhi.* 2014 Sep; 52(9):678–682.

Chevrie-Muller C, Le Normand MT, Forgue M, et al. A peculiar case of acquired aphasia with epilepsy in childhood. *J. Neurolinguist.* 1991; 6:415–431.

Chevrie-Muller C, Narbone J. *Le Langage de l'enfant Aspects et Pathologiques.* 3ème (edn.), Masson, 2007. Spanish (2000) and Portuguese Edition (2005).

Chilosi AM, Brovedani P, Ferrari AR, Ziegler AL, Guerrini R, Deonna T. Language regression associated with autistic regression and electroencephalographic (EEG) abnormalities: A prospective study. *J. Child Neurol.* 2014 Jun; 29(6):855–859.

Chival G, Thibault de Beauregard A. Evaluation du langage oral dans ses aspects structurels et fonctionnels chez six enfants atteints d'épilepsie avec P.O.C.S. (pointes-ondes continues de sommeil). Mémoire. Université Claude-Bernard Lyon I, French, 2000.

Cirelli C, Tononi G. Sleep and synaptic homeostasis sleep. 2015 Jan; 38(1):161–162.

Clarke T, Strug LJ, Murphy PL, et al. High risk of reading disability and speech sound disorder in rolandic epilepsy families: Case-control study. *Epilepsia* 2007 Dec; 48(12):2258–2265.

Cockerell I, Benan N, Bölling G. Landau-Kleffner syndrome. A case study of a 28 year-old woman, Poster: Nordic conference on Rare Diseases in Reykjavik, 2012.

Cockerell I, Bølling G, Nakken KO. Landau-Kleffner syndrome in Norway: Long-term prognosis and experiences with the health services and educational systems. *Epilepsy Behav.* 2011 Jun; 21(2):153–159.

Colamaria V, Sgro V, Caraballo R, et al. Status epilepticus in benign rolandic epilepsy manifesting as anterior operculum syndrome. *Epilepsia* 1991; 32:329–334.

Cole AJ, Andermann F, Taylor L, et al. The Landau-Kleffner syndrome of acquired epileptic aphasia: Unusual clinical outcome, surgical experience, and absence of encephalitis. *Neurology* 1988; 38:31–38.

Connolly AM, Chez M, Streif EM, et al. Brain-derived neurotrophic factor and autoantibodies to neural antigens in sera of children with autistic spectrum disorders, Landau-Kleffner syndrome, and epilepsy. *Biol. Psychiatry.* 2006; 59:354–363.

Connolly AM, Chez MG, Pestronk A, Arnold ST, Mehta S, Deuel RK. Serum autoantibodies to brain in Landau-Kleffner variant, autism, and other neurologic disorders. *J. Pediatr.* 1999; 134:607–613.

Conroy J, McGettigan PA, McCreary D, et al. Towards the identification of a genetic basis for Landau-Kleffner syndrome. *Epilepsia* 2014; 55(6):858–865.

Cooper JA, Ferry PC. Acquired auditory agnosia and seizures in childhood. *J. Speech Hear. Disord.* 1978 May; 43(2):176–184.

Croona C, Kihlgren M, Lundberg S, Eeg-Olofson D, Edebon-Eeg-Olofson K. Neuropsychological findings in children with benign childhood epilepsy with centrotemporal spikes. *Dev. Med. Child Neurol.* 1999; 41:813–818.

References

Cross JH, Neville BG. The surgical treatment of Landau-Kleffner syndrome. *Epilepsia* 2009 Aug; 50(Suppl 7):63–67.

Dalla Bernardina B, Tassinari CA, Dravet C, Bureau M, Beghini G, Roger J. Benign focal epilepsy and "electrical status epilepticus" during sleep (author's transl). *Rev. Electroencephalogr. Neurophysiol. Clin.* 1978 Sep; 8(3):350–353.

Danielsson J, Petermann F. Cognitive deficits in children with benign rolandic epilepsy of childhood or rolandic discharges: A study of children between 4 and 7 years of age with and without seizures compared with healthy controls. *Epilepsy Behav.* 2009 Dec; 16(4):646–651.

Datta AN, Oser N, Bauder F, et al. Cognitive impairment and cortical reorganization in children with benign epilepsy with centrotemporal spikes. *Epilepsia* 2013a Mar; 54(3):487–494.

Datta AN, Oser N, Ramelli GP, et al. BECTS evolving to Landau-Kleffner Syndrome and back by subsequent recovery: a longitudinal language reorganization case study using fMRI, source EEG, and neuropsychological testing. *Epilepsy Behav.* 2013b Apr; 27(1):107–114.

Debiais S, Tuller L, Barthez MA, et al. Epilepsy and language development: The continuous spike-waves during slow sleep syndrome. *Epilepsia* 2007 Jun; 48(6):1104–1110.

Deltour L, Barathon M, Quaglino V, et al. Children with benign epilepsy with centrotemporal spikes (BECTS) show impaired attentional control: evidence from an attentional capture paradigm. *Epileptic Disord.* 2007 Mar; 9(1):32–38.

De Grandis E, Mancardi MM, Carelli V, et al. Epileptic encephalopathy with continuous spike and wave during sleep associated to periventricular leukomalacia. *J. Child. Neurol.* 2014 Nov; 29(11): 1479–1485.

De Negri, M. Electrical status epilepticus during sleep (ESES). Different clinical syndromes: Towards a unifying view? *Brain Dev.* 1997; 19:447–451.

De Negri M, Baglietto MG, Battaglia FM, Gaggero R, Pessagno A, Recanati L. Treatment of electrical status epilepticus by short diazepam (DZP) cycles after DZP rectal bolus test. *Brain Dev.* 1995 Sep–Oct; 17(5):330–333.

Denes G, Balliello S, Volterra V, Pellegrini A. Oral and written language in a case of childhood phonemic deafness. *Brain Lang.* 1986 Nov; 29(2):252–267.

Deonna T. Acquired epileptic aphasia (AEA) or Landau-Kleffner syndrome: From childhood. *Dev. Med. Child Neurol.* 1977; 19:192–207.

Deonna T. Acquired epileptiform aphasia in children (Landau-Kleffner syndrome). *J. Clin. Neurophysiol.* 1991; 8(3):288–298.

Deonna T. Annotation: Cognitive and behavioural correlates of epileptic activity in children. *J. Child. Psychol. Psychiat.* 1993; 34(5):611–620.

Deonna T. Cognitive and behavioral disturbances as epileptic manifestations in children: An overview. *Semin. Pediatr. Neurol.* 1995; 2:254–260.

Deonna T. Epilepsies with cognitive symptomatology. In: Wallace S. (ed.) *Epilepsies in Childhood.* Chapman & Hall Publishers, London, 1996; pp. 315–322.

Deonna T. Developmental consequences of epilepsies in infancy. In: Nehling A, Motte J, Moshé SL, Plouin P. (eds.) *Childhood Epilepsies and Brain Development.* John Libbey, London, 1999; pp. 113–122.

Deonna T. Rolandic epilepsy (RE) - Neuropsychology of the active epilepsy phase. *Epileptic Disord.* 2000a; 2(Suppl 1):S59–S61.

Deonna T. Acquired epileptic aphasia (AEA) or Landau-Kleffner syndrome: From childhood to adulthood. In: Bishop DVM, Leonard LB. (eds.) *Speech and Language Impairments in Children. Causes, Characteristics, Intervention and Outcome.* Psychology Press, Hove, 2000b; pp. 261–272.

Deonna T. Childhood epilepsy: Secondary prevention is crucial. *Dev. Med. Child Neurol.* 2003; 45: 38–41.

Deonna T. Cognitive and behavioral manifestations of epilepsy in children. In: Wallace SJ, Farrell K. (eds.) *Epilepsy in Children.* Arnold, London, 2nd edn., 2004a; pp. 250–256.

Deonna T. Management of epilepsy. Can quality of care be improved? Review. *Arch. Dis. Child.* 2004b; In Press.

Deonna T, Beaumanoir A, Gaillard F, Assal G. Acquired aphasia in childhood with seizure disorder: A heterogeneous syndrome. *Neuropädiatrie* 1977; 8:265–273.

Deonna T, Chevrie C, Hornung E. Childhood epileptic speech disorder: Prolonged, isolated deficit of prosodic features. *Dev. Med. Child Neurol.* 1987; 29:100–105.

173

Deonna T, Davidoff V, Ingvar-Maeder M, Zesiger P, Marcoz JP. The spectrum of cognitive disturbances in children with partial epilepsy and continuous spike waves during sleep. A 4-year follow-up case study with prolonged reversible learning arrest and dysfluency. *Eur. J. Child Neurol.* 1997; 1:19–29.

Deonna T, Davidoff V, Roulet-Perez E. Isolated disturbance of written language acquisition as an initial symptom of epileptic aphasia in a 7 year-old child: A 3-year follow-up study. *Aphasiology* 1993a; 7(5):441–450.

Deonna T, Fletcher P, Voumard C. Temporary regression during language acquisition: A linguistic analysis of a 2 1/2 year-old child. *Dev. Med. Child Neurol.* 1982; 24:156–163.

Deonna, T, Fohlen, M, Jalin C, Delalande O, Ziegler AL. Epileptic stereotypies in children. In: Guerrini R, Aicardi J, Andermann F, Hallett M. (eds.) *Epilepsy and Movement Disorders.* Cambridge University Press, Cambridge, 2002; pp. 319–332.

Deonna T, Peter C, Ziegler AL. Adult follow-up of the acquired aphasia-epilepsy syndrome in childhood. Report of 7 cases. *Neuropediatrics* 1989; 20:132–138.

Deonna T, Prelaz-Girod AC, Mayor-Dubois C, Roulet-Perez E. Sign language in Landau-Kleffner syndrome. *Epilepsia* 2009 Aug; 50(Suppl 7):77–82.

Deonna T, Roulet-Perez E. Acquired epileptic aphasia (AEA): Definition of the syndrome and current problems. In: Beaumanoir A, Bureau M, Deonna T, Mira L, Tassinari CA. (eds.) *Continuous Spikes and Waves during Slow Sleep.* John Libbey, Paris, 1995; pp. 37–45.

Deonna T, Roulet-Perez E. Cognitive and behavioral disorders of epileptic origin in children, *Clinics in Developmental Medicine N0168*, MacKeith Press, 2005.

Deonna T, Roulet-Perez E, Fontan D, Marcoz JP. Speech and oromotor deficits of epileptic origin in benign partial epilepsy of childhood with rolandic spikes (BPERS). Relationship to the acquired aphasia-epilepsy syndrome. *Neuropediatrics* 1993b; 24:83–87.

Deonna T, Roulet-Perez E, Ziegler A.L. Acquired epileptic frontal syndrome in children. In: Beaumanoir A, Andermann F, Mira L, Zifkin B. (eds.) *Frontal Lobe Seizures and Epilepsies in Children.* John Libbey, Montrouge, France, 2003.

Deonna T, Roulet-Perez E. Early-onset acquired epileptic aphasia (Landau-Kleffner syndrome, LKS) and regressive autistic disorders with epileptic EEG abnormalities: The continuing debate. *Brain Dev.* 2010 Oct; 32(9):746–752.

Deonna T, Roulet-Perez E, Cronel-Ohayon S, Mayor-Dubois C. Correspondence on "deterioration in cognitive function in children with benign epilepsy of childhood with central temporal spikes treated with sulthiame". *J. Child Neurol.* 2010 Jan; 25(1):127–128.

Deonna T, Ziegler AL. Hypothalamic hamartoma, precocious puberty and gelastic seizures: A special model of "epileptic" developmental disorder. *Epileptic Disord.* 2000; 2:33–37.

Deonna T, Zesiger P, Davidoff V, Maeder M, Mayor C, Roulet-Perez E. Benign partial epilepsy of childhood: A neuropsychological and EEG study of cognitive function. *Dev. Med. Child. Neurol.* 2000; 42:595–603.

Deonna T, Ziegler AL, Maeder IM, Ansermet F, Roulet-Perez E. Reversible behavioural autistic-like regression: A manifestation of a special (new?) epileptic syndrome in a 28-month-old child. A 2-year longitudinal study. *Neurocase* 1995; 1:91–99.

Deonna T, Ziegler AL, Moura-Serra J, Innocenti G. Autistic regression in relation to limbic pathology and epilepsy: Report of two cases. *Dev. Med. Child Neurol.* 1993c; 35:166–176.

De Rose P, Perrino F, Lettori D, et al. Visual and visuoperceptual function in children with Panayiotopoulos syndrome. *Epilepsia* 2010 Jul; 51(7):1205–1211.

De Saint-Martin A, Petiau C, Massa R, et al. Idiopathic rolandic epilepsy with "interictal" facial myoclonia and oromotor deficit: A longitudinal EEG and PET study. *Epilepsia* 1999; 40(5):614–620.

De Tiège X, Goldman S, Laureys S, et al. Regional cerebral glucose metabolism in epilepsies with continuous spikes and waves during sleep. *Neurology* 2004; 63:853–857.

De Tiège X, Goldman S, Van Bogaert P. Insights into the pathophysiology of psychomotor regression in CSWS syndromes from FDG-PET and EEG-fMRI. *Epilepsia* 2009; 50(Suppl 7):47–50.

De Tiège X, Goldman S, Van Bogaert P. Neuronal networks in children with continuous spikes and waves during slow sleep. *Brain* 2011; 134:e177.

De Tiège X, Goldman S, Verheulpen D, Aeby A, Poznanski N, Van Bogaert P, et al. Coexistence of idiopathic rolandic epilepsy and CSWS in two families. *Epilepsia* 2006; 47:1723–1727.

De Tiège X, Harrison S, Laufs H, et al. Impact of interictal epileptic activity on normal brain function in epileptic encephalopathy: An electroencephalography-functional magnetic resonance imaging study. *Epilepsy Behav.* 2007 Nov; 11(3):460–465.

References

De Tiège X, Ligot N, Goldman S, et al. Metabolic evidence for remote inhibition in epilepsies with continuous spike-waves during sleep. *Neuroimage* 2008; 40:802–810.

De Tiège X, Trotta N, Op de Beeck M, et al. Neurophysiological activity underlying altered brain metabolism in epileptic encephalopathies with CSWS. *Epilepsy Res.* 2013; 105:316–325.

Diagnostic and Statistical Manual of Mental Disorders, 4th edition. Wahington DC: American Psychiatric Association, 1994.

Diagnostic and Statistical Manual of Mental Disorders, 5th edition. Wahington DC: American Psychiatric Association, 2013.

Dibbens LM, de Vries B, Donatello S, et al. Mutations in DEPDC5 cause familial focal epilepsy with variable foci. *Nat Genet.* 2013 May; 45(5):546–551.

Doherty CP, Fitzsimons M, Asenbauer B, et al. Prosodic preservation in Landau-Kleffner syndrome: A case report. *Eur. J. Neurol.* 1999 Mar; 6(2):227–234.

Dong C, Sriram S, Delbeke D, et al. Aphasic or amnesic status epilepticus detected on PET but not EEG. *Epilepsia* 2009; 50:251–255.

Doose H, Bayer WK, Ernst JP, Tuxhorn I, Volzke E. Benign partial epilepsy. Treatment with sulthiame. *Dev. Med. Child Neurol.* 1988; 30:683–684.

Doose H, Neubauer B, Carlsson G. Children with benign focal sharp waves in the EEG - Developmental disorders and epilepsy. *Neuropediatrics* 1996; 27:227–241.

Downes M, Greenaway R, Clark M, et al. Outcome following multiple subpial transection in Landau-Kleffner syndrome and related regression. *Epilepsia* 2015 Nov; 56(11):1760–1766.

Dugas M, Masson M, Le Heuzey MF, Regnier N. Childhood acquired aphasia with epilepsy (Landau-Kleffner syndrome). 12 personal cases. *Rev. Neurol. (Paris)* 1982; 138(10):755–780.

Dulac O, Billard C, Arthuis M. Aspects electrocliniques et évolutifs de l'épilepsie dans le syndrome aphasie-épilepsie. *Arch. Fr. Pediatr.* 1983; 40:299–308.

Duncan JS. Imaging and epilepsy. *Brain* 1997; 120:339–377.

Duvelleroy-Hommel C, Billard C, Lucas P, et al. Sleep EEG and developmental dysphasia: Lack of a consistent relationship with paroxysmal EEG activity during sleep. *Neuropediatrics* 1995; 26(1):14–18.

Echenne B, Cheminal R, Rivier F, Negre C, Touchon J, Billiard M. Epileptic encephalopathic abnormalities and developmental dysphasias: A study of 32 patients. *Brain Dev.* 1992; 14:216–225.

Endele S, Rosenberger G, Geider K, et al. Mutations in GRIN2A and GRIN2B encoding regulatory subunits of NMDA receptors cause variable neurodevelopmental phenotypes. *Nat. Genet.* 2010 Nov; 42(11):1021–1026.

Engel J. Report of the ILAE Classification Core Group. *Epilepsia* 2006; 47:1558–1568.

Engler F, Maeder-Ingvar M, Roulet-Perez E, Deonna T. Treatment with Sulthiame (Ospolot®) in benign partial epilepsy of childhood and related syndromes: An open clinical and EEG study. *Neuropediatrics* 2003; 34:105–109.

Ewen JB, Vining EP, Smith CA, et al. Cognitive and EEG fluctuation in benign childhood epilepsy with central-temporal spikes: a case series. *Epilepsy Res.* 2011 Nov; 97(1–2):214–219.

Fattinger S, Schmitt B, Bölsterli Heinzle BK, Critelli H, Jenni OG, Huber R. Impaired slow wave sleep downscaling in patients with infantile spasms. *Eur. J. Paediatr Neurol.* 2015 Mar; 19(2):134–142.

Feekery CJ, Parry-Fielder B, Hopkins IJ. Landau-Kleffner syndrome: Six patients including discordant monozygotic twins. *Pediatr. Neurol.* 1993 Jan–Feb; 9(1):49–53.

Fejerman N. Atypical rolandic epilepsy. *Epilepsia* 2009 Aug; 50 (Suppl 7):9–12.

Fejerman N, Caraballo R, Cersósimo R, Ferraro SM, Galicchio S, Amartino H. Sulthiame add-on therapy in children with focal epilepsies associated with encephalopathy related to electrical status epilepticus during slow sleep (ESES). *Epilepsia* 2012 Jul; 53(7):1156–1161.

Fejerman N, Caraballo R, Tenembaum SN. Atypical evolutions of benign localization-related epilepsies in children: Are they predictable? *Epilepsia* 2000; 41(4):380–390.

Filippini M, Ardu E, Stefanelli S, Boni A, Gobbi G, Benso F. Neuropsychological profile in new-onset benign epilepsy with centrotemporal spikes (BECTS): Focusing on executive functions. *Epilepsy Behav.* 2016 Jan; 54:71–79.

Filippini M, Boni A, Giannotta M, Gobbi G. Neuropsychological development in children belonging to BECTS spectrum: Long-term effect of epileptiform activity. *Epilepsy Behav.* 2013 Sep; 28(3):504–511.

Fine A. Nickels K2 Temporoparietal resection in a patient with Landau-Kleffner syndrome. *Semin. Pediatr. Neurol.* 2014 Jun; 21(2):96–100.

Frank. Why I am not SHY: a reply to Tononi and Cirelli, *Neural Plasticity* 2013.

Frith CD, Frith U. Social cognition in humans. *Curr. Biol.* 2007; 17(16):R724–R732.

175

Gaillard WD, Weinstein S, Conry J, et al. Prognosis of children with partial epilepsy: MRI and serial 18FDG-PET. *Neurology* 2007; 68:655–659.

Galer S, Urbain C, De Tiège X, et al. Impaired sleep-related consolidation of declarative memories in idiopathic focal epilepsies of childhood. *Epilepsy Behav.* 2015 Feb; 43:16–23.

Gallagher S, Weiss S, Oram Cardy J, Humphries T, Harman KE, Menascu S. Efficacy of very high dose steroid treatment in a case of Landau-Kleffner syndrome. *Dev. Med. Child Neurol.* 2006 Sep; 48(9):766–769.

Gascon G, Victor D, Lombroso CT. Language disorders, convulsive disorder, and electroencephalographic abnormalities. Acquired syndrome in children. *Arch. Neurol.* 1973 Mar; 28(3):156–162.

Genizi J, Shamay-Tsoory SG, Shahar E, Yaniv S, Aharon-Perez J. Impaired social behavior in children with benign childhood epilepsy with centrotemporal spikes. *J Child Neurol.* 2012 Feb; 27(2):156–161.

Glos J, Jariabkova K, Szabova I. Landau-Kleffner syndrome: A case of a dissociation between spoken and written language. *Bratisl. Lek. Listy.* 2001; 102(12):556–561.

Gobbi G, Boni A, Filippini M. The spectrum of idiopathic Rolandic epilepsy syndromes and idiopathic occipital epilepsies: From the benign to the disabling. *Epilepsia* 2006; 47(Suppl 2):62–66.

Gotts SJ, Simmons WK, Milbury LA, Wallace GL, Cox RW, Martin A. Fractionation of social brain circuits in autism spectrum disorders. *Brain.* 2012 Sep; 135(Pt 9):2711–2725.

Grosjean F. Living with two languages. In: Paranlis I. (ed.) *Cultural and Language Diversity and the Deaf Experience.* Cambridge University Press, Cambridge, 1996; pp. 20–37.

Gross-Selbeck G. Treatment of "benign" partial epilepsies of childhood, including atypical forms. *Neuropediatrics* 1995 Feb; 26(1):45–50.

Grote CL, Van Slyke P, Hoeppner JA. Language outcome following multiple subpial transection for Landau-Kleffner syndrome. *Brain* 1999 Mar; 122(Pt 3):561–566.

Gubser-Mercati D, Mayor-Dubois C, Deonna T, Roulet-Perez E. Primary neonatal thalamic haemorrhage and epilepsy with continuous spike-waves during sleep(CSWS). Early acquired steroid responsive severe attention deficit disorder *Europ. J. Ped Neurol.* Abstract, 2005.

Gusnard DA, Raichle ME. Searching for a baseline: Functional imaging and the resting human brain. *Nat. Rev. Neurosci.* 2001; 2:685–694.

Guzzetta F, Battaglia D, Veredice C, et al. Early thalamic injury associated with epilepsy and continuous spike-wave during slow sleep. *Epilepsia* 2005 Jun; 46(6):889–900.

Hahn A, Pistohl J, Neubauer BA, Stephani U. Atypical "benign" partial epilepsy or pseudo-Lennox-syndrome – Clinical symptomatology and long-term prognosis. *Neuropediatrics* 2001; 32(1):9–13.

Halász P, Kelemen A, Clemens B, et al. The perisylvian epileptic network. A unifying concept. *Ideggyogy Sz.* 2005 Jan 20; 58(1–2):21–31.

Hämäläinen M, Hari R, Ilmoniemi RJ, Knuutila J, Lounasmaa OV. Magnetoencephalography: Theory, instrumentation, and applications to noninvasive studies of the working human brain. *Rev. Mod. Phys.* 1993; 65:413–497.

Handforth A, Finch DM, Peters R, Tan AM, Treiman DM. Interictal spiking increases 2-deoxy[14C]glucose uptake and c-fos-like reactivity. *Ann. Neurol.* 1994; 35:724–731.

Heller T. Uber Dementia Infantilis. *Ztschr. Erforsh. Behandl. Jugendl. Schwachsinns.* 1908; 2:17–28.

Hickok G. The functional neuroanatomy of language. *Phys. Life Rev.* 2009 Sep; 6(3):121–143.

Hickok G. The cortical organization of speech processing: Feedback control and predictive coding the context of a dual-stream model. *J. Comm. Disord.* 2012 Nov–Dec; 45(6):393–402.

Hickok G, Poeppel D. The cortical organization of speech processing. *Nat. Rev.* 2007; 8:393–402.

Hirsch E, Marescaux C, Maquet P, et al. Landau-Kleffner syndrome: A clinical and EEG study of 5 cases. *Epilepsia* 1990; 31:768–777.

Holmes GL, McKeever M, Saunders Z. Epileptiform activity in aphasia of childhood: An epiphenomenon? *Epilepsia* 1981 Dec; 22(6):631–639.

Holmes GL, Lenck-Santini PP. Role of interictal epileptiform abnormalities in cognitive impairment. *Epilepsy Behav.* 2006 May; 8(3):504–515.

Hommet C, Billard C, Motte J, et al. Cognitive function in adolescents and young adults in complete remission from benign childhood epilepsy with centro-temporal spikes. *Epileptic Disord.* 2001 Dec; 3(4):207–216.

Huber R, Ghilardi MF, Massimini M, Tononi G. Local sleep and learning. *Nature* 2004; 430:78–81.

Huppke P, Kallenberg K, Gärtner J. Perisylvian polymicrogyria in Landau-Kleffner syndrome. *Neurology* 2005 May; 64(9):1660.

Iadecola C, Nedergaard M. Glial regulation of the cerebral microvasculature. *Nat. Neurosci.* 2007; 10:1369–1376.

References

ILAE. Proposal for revised classification of Epilepsies and Epileptic Syndromes. *Epilepsia* 1989; 30(4):389–399.

Irwin K, Birch V, Lees J, et al. Multiple subpial transection in Landau-Kleffner syndrome. *Dev. Med. Child Neurol.* 2001 Apr; 43(4):248–252.

Issa NP. Neurobiology of continuous spike-wave in slow-wave sleep and Landau-Kleffner syndromes. *Pediatr Neurol.* 2014 Sep; 51(3):287–296.

Jakab I. L'aphasie dans la démence infantile de Heller. *Encéphale* 1950; 39(3):220–253.

Jokeit H, Seitz RJ, Markowitsch HJ, Neumann N, Witte OW, Ebner A. Prefrontal asymmetric interictal glucose hypometabolism and cognitive impairment in patients with temporal lobe epilepsy. *Brain* 1997; 120:2283–2294.

Jurkevičienė G, Endzinienė M, Laukienė I, et al. Association of language dysfunction and age of onset of benign epilepsy with centrotemporal spikes in children. *Eur. J. Paediatr Neurol.* 2012 Nov; 16(6):653–661.

Kaga M. Language disorders in Landau-Kleffner syndrome. *J. Child Neurol.* 1999 Feb; 14(2):118–122.

Kaga M, Inagaki M, Ohta R. Epidemiological study of Landau-Kleffner syndrome (LKS) in Japan. *Brain Dev.* 2014 Apr; 36(4):284–286.

Kallay C, Mayor-Dubois C, Maeder-Ingvar M, et al. Reversible acquired epileptic frontal syndrome and CSWS suppression in a child with congenital hemiparesis treated by hemispherotomy. *Eur. J. Paediatr. Neurol.* 2009 Sep; 13(5):430–438.

Kasteleijn-Nolst Trenité DGA, Siebelink BM, Berends SCG, Van Strien JW, Meinardi H. Lateralited effects of subclinical epileptiform EEG discharges on scholastic performance in children. *Epilepsia* 1990b; 31(6):740–745.

Kasteleijn-Nolst Trenité DGA, Smit AM, Velis DN, Willemse J, van Emde Boas W. On-line detection of transient neuropsychological disturbances during EEG discharges in children with epilepsy. *Dev. Med. Child Neurol.* 1990a Jan; 32(1):46–50.

Kersbergen KJ, de Vries LS, Leijten FS, et al. Neonatal thalamic hemorrhage is strongly associated with electrical status epilepticus in slow wave sleep. *Epilepsia* 2013 Apr; 54(4):733–740.

Kim-Dufor D-H, Ferragne E, Dufor O, Astésano C, Nespoulous J.L. A novel prosody assessment test: Findings in three cases of Landau-Kleffner syndrome. *J. Neurolinguist.* 2012; 25(3):1–18.

Kong J, Shepel PN, Holden CP, Mackiewicz M, Pack AI, Geiger JD. Brain glycogen decreases with increased periods of wakefulness: Implications for homeostatic drive to sleep. *J. Neurosci.* 2002; 22:5581–5587.

Korkman M, Granström ML, Appelqvist K, Liukkonen E. Neuropsychological characteristics of five children with the Landau-Kleffner syndrome: Dissociation of auditory and phonological discrimination. *J. Int. Neuropsychol. Soc.* 1998; 4:566–575.

Koupernik C. Conséquences d'un attentat sexuel chez une fillette de 4 ans. *La psychiatrie de l'enfant* 1969; 12(1):267–298.

Koupernik C, Masciangelo PM, Balestra-Beretta S. A case of Heller's dementia following sexual assault in a four year old girl. *Child Psychiatry Hum. Dev.* 1972; 2(3):134–144.

Kramer U, Ben-Zeev B, Harel S, Kivity S. Transient oromotor deficits in children with benign childhood epilepsy with central temporal spikes. *Epilepsia* 2001; 42(5):616–620.

Kubota M, Takeshita K, Saitoh M, Hirose H, Kimura I, Sakakihara Y. Magnetoencephalographic analysis of rolandic discharges in a patient with rolandic epilepsy associated with oromotor deficits. *J. Child Neurol.* 2004; 19:456–459.

Kugler SL, Bali B, Lieberman P, et al. An autosomal dominant genetically heterogeneous variant of rolandic epilepsy and speech disorder. *Epilepsia* 2008 Jun; 49(6):1086–1090.

Kuzniecky R, Andermann F, Guerrini R. Congenital bilateral perisylvian syndrome: Study of 31 patients. The CBPS Multicenter Collaborative Study. *Lancet* 1993 Mar; 341(8845):608–612.

Kwon S, Seo HE, Hwang SK. Cognitive and other neuropsychological profiles in children with newly diagnosed benign rolandic epilepsy. *Korean J Pediatr.* 2012 Oct; 55(10):383–387.

Kyllerman M, Nyden A, Prauin N, Rasmussen P, Wetterquist AK, Hedström A. Transient psychosis in a girl with epilepsy and continuous spikes and waves during slow sleep (CSWS). *Eur. Child Adoles. Psychiatry* 1996; 5(4):216–221.

Lagae LG, Silberstein J, Gillis PL, Casaer PJ. Successful use of intravenous immunoglobulins in Landau-Kleffner syndrome. *Pediatr. Neurol.* 1998; 18(2):165–168.

Lahnakoski JM, Glerean E, Salmi J, et al. Naturalistic FMRI mapping reveals superior temporal sulcus as the hub for the distributed brain network for social perception. *Front. Hum. Neurosci.* 13 Aug 2012; 6:233.

Lal D, Pernhorst K, Klein KM, et al. Extending the phenotypic spectrum of RBFOX1 deletions: Sporadic focal epilepsy. *Epilepsia* 2015 Sep; 56(9):e129–e133.

Landau WM, Kleffner FR. Syndrome of acquired aphasia with convulsive disorder in children. *Neurology* 1957; 7:523–530.

Lane HL. *The Mask of Benevolence: Disabling the Deaf Community.* Vintage Books, New York, 1993; p. 132.

Lanzi G, Veggiotti P, Conte S, Partesana E, Resi C. A correlated fluctuation of language and EEG abnormalities in a case of the Landau-Kleffner syndrome. *Brain Dev.* 1994 Jul–Aug; 16(4):329–334.

Larrieu JL, Lagueny A, Ferrer X, Julien J. [Epilepsy with continuous discharges during slow-wave sleep. Treatment with clobazam]. *Rev. Electroencephalogr. Neurophysiol. Clin.* 1986 Dec; 16(4):383–394.

Leal AJ, Ferreira JC, Dias AI, Calado E. Origin of frontal lobe spikes in the early onset benign occipital lobe epilepsy (Panayiotopoulos syndrome). *Clin. Neurophysiol.* 2008 Sep; 119(9):1985–1991.

Lemke JR, Lal D, Reinthaler EM, et al. Mutations in GRIN2A cause idiopathic focal epilepsy with rolandic spikes. *Nat. Genet.* 2013; 45:1067–1072.

Lengler U, Kafadar I, Neubauer BA, Krakow K. fMRI correlates of interictal epileptic activity in patients with idiopathic benign focal epilepsy of childhood. A simultaneous EEG-functional MRI study. *Epilepsy Res.* 2007; 75:29–38.

Leppänen JM, Nelson CA. Tuning the developing brain to social signals of emotions. *Nat. Rev. Neurosci.* 2009 Jan; 10(1):37–47.

Lerman P, Lerman-Sagie T, Kivity S. Effect of early corticosteroid therapy for Landau-Kleffner syndrome. *Dev. Med. Child Neurol.* 1991 Mar; 33(3):257–260.

Lesca G, Rudolf G, Bruneau N, et al. GRIN2A mutations in acquired epileptic aphasia and related childhood focal epilepsies and encephalopathies with speech and language dysfunction. *Nat. Genet.* 2013; 45:1061–1066.

Lévêque Y, Deonna T, Mayor-Dubois C, Roulet-Perez E, Caclin A, Tillmann B. Deficits in music processing in Landau-Kleffner syndrome: case studies in adulthood. In preparation, 2016.

Lewine JD, Andrews R, Chez M, et al. Magnetoencephalographic patterns of epileptiform activity in children with regressive autism spectrum disorders. *Pediatrics* 1999 Sep; 104(3 Pt 1):405–418.

Liberman AM. Some results of research on speech perception. *Journal of the Acoustic Society of America* 1957; 29(1):117–123.

Ligot N, Archambaud F, Trotta N, et al. Default mode network hypometabolism in epileptic encephalopathies with CSWS. *Epilepsy Res.* 2014; 108:861–871.

Lillywhite LM, Saling MM, Harvey AS, et al. Neuropsychological and functional MRI studies provide converging evidence of anterior language dysfunction in BECTS. *Epilepsia* 2009 Oct; 50(10):2276–2284.

Lindgren S, Kihlgren M, Melin L, Croona C, Lundberg S, Eeg-Olofsson O. Development of cognitive functions in children with rolandic epilepsy. *Epilepsy Behav.* 2004 Dec; 5(6):903–910.

Liukkonen E, Kantola-Sorsa E, Paetau R, Gaily E, Peltola M, Granström ML. Long-term outcome of 32 children with encephalopathy with status epilepticus during sleep, or ESES syndrome. *Epilepsia* 2010 Oct; 51(10):2023–2032.

Loiseau P, Cohadon F, Mortureux Y. A propos d'une forme singulière d'épilepsie de l'enfant. *Rev. Neurol.* 1967; 116(3):244–248.

Loiseau P, Pestre M, Dartigues JF, Commenges D, Berbeyer-Gateau C, Cohadon S. Long-term prognosis in two forms of childhood epilepsy: Typical absence seizures and epilepsy with Rolandic (centrotemporal) EEG foci. *Ann. Neurol.* 1983; 13:642–648.

Lombroso CT. Sylvian seizures and midtemporal spike foci in children. *Arch. Neurol.* 1967 Jul; 17(1):52–59.

Lopes R, Simões MR, Leal AJ. Neuropsychological abnormalities in children with the Panayiotopoulos syndrome point to parietal lobe dysfunction. *Epilepsy Behav.* 2014 Feb; 31:50–55.

Losito E, Battaglia D, Chieffo D, et al. Sleep-potentiated epileptiform activity in early thalamic injuries: Study in a large series (60 cases). *Epilepsy Res.* 2015 Jan; 109:90–99.

Lou HC, Brandt S, Bruhn P. Aphasia and epilepsy in childhood. *Acta Neurol. Scand.* 1977 Jul; 56(1):46–54.

Luat AF, Chugani HT, Asano E, Juhász C, Trock G, Rothermel R. Episodic receptive aphasia in a child with Landau-Kleffner Syndrome: PET correlates. *Brain Dev.* 2006 Oct; 28(9):592–596.

Lugaresi E. L'afasia nelle regression infantile; considerazioni a proposito di un caso. *Riv. Sper. Freniatr. Med. Leg. Alien. Ment.* 1958; 82(4):935–948.

Lundberg S, Eeg-Olofsson O, Raininko R, Eeg-Olofsson KE. Hippocampal asymmetries and white matter abnormalities on MRI in benign childhood epilepsy with centrotemporal spikes. *Epilepsia* 1999 Dec; 40(12):1808–1815.

Lundberg S, Frylmark A, Eeg-Olofsson O. Children with rolandic epilepsy have abnormalities of oromotor and dichotic listening performance. *Dev. Med. Child Neurol.* 2005; 47(9):603–608.

References

Maccario M, Hefferen SJ, Keblusek SJ, Lipinski KA. Developmental dysphasia and electroencephalographic abnormalities. *Dev. Med. Child Neurol.* 1982; 24(2):141–155.

MacSweeney M, Capek CM, Campbell R, Woll B. The signing brain: the neurobiology of sign language. *Trends Cogn Sci.* 2008 Nov; 12(11):432–440.

Magistretti PJ. Neuron-glia metabolic coupling and plasticity. *J. Exp. Biol.* 2006; 209:2304–2311.

Majerus S, Laureys S, Collette F, et al. Phonological short-term memory networks following recovery from Landau-Kleffner syndrome. *Hum. Brain Mapp.* 2003; 19(3):133–144.

Majerus S, Van der Linden M, Poncelet M, Metz-Lutz MN. Can phonological and semantic short-term memory be dissociated? Further evidence from Landau-Kleffner syndrome. *Cogn. Neuropsychol.* 2004; 21(5):491–512.

Mantovani JF, Landau WM. Acquired aphasia with convulsive disorder: Course and prognosis. *Neurology* 1980; 30:524–529.

Maquet P, Hirsch E, Metz-Lutz MN, et al. Regional cerebral glucose metabolism in children with deterioration of one or more cognitive functions and continuous spike-and-wave discharges during sleep. *Brain* 1995; 118:1497–1520.

Marescaux C, Hirsch E, Finck S. Landau-Kleffner syndrome: A pharmacological study of 5 cases. *Epilepsia* 1990; 31:768–777.

Mariën P, Saerens J, Verslegers W, Borggreve F, De Deyn PP. Some controversies about type and nature of aphasic symptomatology in Landau-Kleffner's syndrome: A case study. *Acta Neurol. Belg.* 1993; 93(4):183–203.

Mariën P, Verhoeven J, Wackenier P, Engelborghs S, De Deyn PP. Foreign accent syndrome as a developmental motor speech disorder. *Cortex* 2009 Jul–Aug; 45(7):870–878.

Marshall J, Atkinson J, Woll B, Thacker A. Aphasia in a bilingual user of British sign language and English: Effects of cross-linguistic cues( ). *Cogn. Neuropsychol.* 2005 Sep; 22(6):719–736.

Marshall JC. Signs of language in the brain. *Nature* 1986 Jul 24–30; 322(6077):307–308.

Martín Miguel Mdel C, García Seoane JJ, Valentín A, et al. EEG latency analysis for hemispheric lateralisation in Landau-Kleffner syndrome. *Clin. Neurophysiol.* 2011 Feb; 122(2):244–252.

Massa R, de Saint-Martin A, Carcangiu R, et al. EEG criteria predictive of complicated evolution in idiopathic rolandic epilepsy. *Neurology* 2001; 57(6):1071–1079.

Masterton RA, Harvey AS, Archer JS, et al. Focal epileptiform spikes do not show a canonical BOLD response in patients with benign rolandic epilepsy (BECTS). *Neuroimage* 2010; 51:252–260.

Matricardi S, Deleo F, Ragona F, et al. Neuropsychological profiles and outcomes in children with new onset frontal lobe epilepsy. *Epilepsy Behav.* 2016 Feb; 55:79–83.

Matsui T, Ishikawa T, Ito H, et al. Brain glycogen supercompensation following exhaustive exercise. *J. Physiol.* 2012; 590:607–616.

Mayor Dubois C, Gianella D, Chaves-Vischer V, Haenggeli CA, Deonna T, Roulet-Perez E. Speech delay due to a prelinguitic regression of epileptic origin. *Neuropediatrics* 2004; 35:50–53.

Mayor Dubois C, Zesiger P, Roulet-Perez E, Maeder-Ingvar M, Deonna T. Acquired epileptic dysgraphia: A longitudinal study. *Dev. Med. Child Neurol.* 2003; 45:807–812.

McKinney W, McGreal DA. An aphasic syndrome in children. *Can. Med. Assoc. J.* 1974 Mar; 110(6): 637–639.

McVicar KA, Ballaban-Gil K, Rapin I, Moshé SL, Shinnar S. Epileptiform EEG abnormalities in children with language regression. *Neurology* 2005 Jul; 65(1):129–131.

Menkes JH. *Textbook of Child Neurology*. Lea & Febiger, Philadelphia, London, 1974; 1st edn.

Menkes JH. *Textbook of Child Neurology*. Williams & Wilkins, Baltimore, Maryland, 1995.

Metz-Lutz MN. The assessment of auditory function in CSWS: Lessons from long-term outcome. *Epilepsia* 2009 Aug; 50(Suppl 7):73–76.

Metz-Lutz MN, Hirsch E, Maquet P, et al. Dichotic Listening Performances in the follow-up of Landau-Kleffner syndrome. *Child Neuropsychology* 1997; 3(1):47–60.

Metz-Lutz MN, Kleitz C, De Saint-Martin A, Massa R, Hirsch E, Marescaux C. Cognitive development in benign focal epilepsies of childhood. *Dev. Neurosci.* 1999; 21(3–5):182–190.

Metz-Lutz MN, Maquet P, de Saint Martin A, et al. Pathophysiological aspects of Landau-Kleffner syndrome: From the active epileptic phase to recovery. *Int. Rev. Neurobiol.* 2001; 45:505–526.

Meyer Mercer. Frog.Where are you?. Sequel to a boy, a dog and a frog. Dial Books for Young Readers, Piered piper book, New York.

Mikati MA, El-Bitar MK, Najjar MW, et al. A child with refractory complex partial seizures, right temporal ganglioglioma, contralateral continuous electrical status epilepticus, and a secondary Landau-Kleffner autistic syndrome. *Epilepsy Behav.* 2009 Feb; 14(2):411–417.

Mikati MA, Saab R, Fayad MN, Choueiri RN. Efficacy of intravenous immunoglobulin in Landau-Kleffner syndrome. *Pediatr. Neurol.* 2002 Apr; 26(4):298–300.

Moeller F, Moehring J, Ick I, et al. EEG-fMRI in atypical benign partial epilepsy. *Epilepsia* 2013; 54:e103–e108.

Monjauze C, Broadbent H, Boyd SG, Neville BG, Baldeweg T. Language deficits and altered hemispheric lateralization in young people in remission from BECTS. *Epilepsia* 2011 Aug; 52(8):e79–e83.

Monteiro JP, Roulet-Perez E, Davidoff V, Deonna T. Primary neonatal thalamic haemorrhage and epilepsy with continuous spike-wave during sleep: A longitudinal follow-up of a possible significant relation. *Eur. J. Paediatr. Neurol.* 2001; 5:41–47.

Montford M, Sanchez A. L'intervention dans les troubles graves de l'acquisition du langage et les dysphasies développementales Editeur: Ortho Edition, 2007.

Morrell F, Whisler WW, Bleck TP. Multiple subpial transection: A new approach to the surgical treatment of focal epilepsy. *J. Neurosurg.* 1989 Feb; 70(2):231–239.

Morrell F, Whisler WW, Smith MC, et al. Landau-Kleffner syndrome: Treatment with subpial intracortical transection. *Brain* 1995; 118:1529–1546.

Mulas F. (ed.) *Trastornos del Lenguaje en la Infancia.* Barcelona, Spain: Viquera Editores, 2013.

Nass R, Devinsky O. Autistic regression with rolandic spikes. *Neuropsychiatry Neuropsychol. Behav. Neurol.* 1999a; 12(3):193–197.

Nass R, Gross A, Devinsky O. Autism and autistic epileptiform regression with occipital spikes. *Dev. Med. Child Neurol.* 1998; 40:453–458.

Nass R, Gross A, Wisoff J, Devinsky O. Outcome of multiple subpial transections for autistic epileptiform regression. *Pediatr. Neurol.* 1999b; 21(1):464–470.

Nation JE, Dorothy MA. *Diagnosis of Speech and Language Disorders.* College-Hill Press, San Diego, CA, 1984.

Nelissen N, Van Paesschen W, Baete K, et al. Correlations of interictal FDG-PET metabolism and ictal SPECT perfusion changes in human temporal lobe epilepsy with hippocampal sclerosis. *Neuroimage* 2006; 32:684–695.

Neri ML, Guimarães CA, Oliveira EP, et al. Neuropsychological assessment of children with rolandic epilepsy: executive functions. *Epilepsy Behav.* 2012 Aug; 24(4):403–407.

Neuschlová L, Sterbová K, Zácková J, Komárek V. Epileptiform activity in children with developmental dysphasia: Quantification of discharges in overnight sleep video-EEG. *Epileptic Disord.* 2007 Dec; 9(Suppl 1):S28–S35.

Neville BGR, Burch V, Cass H, Lees J. Behavioural aspects of Landau-Kleffner syndrome. *Clin. Dev. Med.* 2000; 149:56–63.

Neville BGR, Burch V, Cass H, Lees J. Motor disorders in Landau-Kleffner syndrome(LKS). *Epilepsia* 1998; 39(Suppl 6):123.

Neville BGR, Harkness WF, Cross JH, et al. Surgical treatment of severe autistic regression in childhood epilepsy. *Pediatr Neurol.* 1997; 16(2):137–140.

Nevsimalova S, Tauberova A, Doutlik S, Kucera V, Dlouha O. A role of autoimmunity in the etiopathogenesis of Landau-Kleffner syndrome. *Brain Dev.* 1992; 14:342–345.

Nickels K, Wirrell E. Electrical status epilepticus in sleep. *Semin. Pediatr. Neurol.* 2008 Jun; 15(2):50–60.

Nikanorova M, Miranda MJ, Atkins M, Sahlholdt L. Ketogenic diet in the treatment of refractory continuous spikes and waves during slow sleep. *Epilepsia* 2009 May; 50(5):1127–1131.

Northcott E, Connolly AM, Berroya A, et al. The neuropsychological and language profile of children with benign rolandic epilepsy. *Epilepsia* 2005 Jun; 46(6):924–930.

Novartis Found Symp. Book series No 251: Autism: Neural basis and treatment possibilities, Wiley, Chichester ed. See final discussion (Frith, Happé, Folstein) 2003; 281–288.

Novotny EJ Jr, Fulbright RK, Pearl PL, Gibson KM, Rothman DL. Magnetic resonance spectroscopy of neurotransmitters in human brain. *Ann. Neurol.* 2003; 54(Suppl 6):S25–S31.

Ntsambi-Eba G, Vaz G, Docquier MA, van Rijckevorsel K, Raftopoulos C. Patients with refractory epilepsy treated using a modified multiple subpial transection technique. *Neurosurgery* 2013 Jun; 72(6):890–897.

Otero E, Cordova S, Diaz F, Garcia-Teruel I, Del Brutto OH. Acquired epileptic aphasia (the Landau-Kleffner syndrome) due to neurocysticercosis. *Epilepsia* 1989 Sep–Oct; 30(5):569–572.

Paetau R. Magnetoencephalography in Landau-Kleffner syndrome. *Epilepsia* 2009 Aug; 50(Suppl 7):51–54.

Pal DK. Epilepsy and neurodevelopmental disorders of language. *Curr. Opin. Neurol.* 2011 Apr; 24(2):126–131.

Pan A, Luders HO. Epileptiform discharges in benign focal epilepsy of childhood. *Epileptic Disord.* 2000; 2(Suppl 1):S29–S36.

Panayotopoulos CP. *Benign Childhood Partial Seizures and Related Epileptic Syndromes.* John Libbey, London, 1999.

References

Papagno C, Basso A. Impairment of written language and mathematic skills in a case of Landau-Kleffner syndrome. *Aphasiology* 1993; 7(5):541–561.

Paquier PF, Verheulpen D, De Tiège X, Van Bogaert P. Acquired cognitive dysfunction with focal sleep spiking activity. *Epilepsia* 2009 Aug; 50(Suppl 7):29–32.

Park YD. The effects of vagus nerve stimulation therapy on patients with intractable seizures and either Landau-Kleffner syndrome or autism. *Epilepsy Behav.* 2003 Jun; 4(3):286–290.

Pardoe HR, Berg AT, Archer JS, Fulbright RK, Jackson GD. A neurodevelopmental basis for BECTS: Evidence from structural MRI. *Epilepsy Res.* 2013 Jul; 105(1–2):133–139.

Parry-Fielder B, Collins K, Fisher J, et al. Electroencephalographic abnormalities during sleep in children with developmental speech-language disorders: A case-control study. *Dev. Med. Child Neurol.* 2009 Mar; 51(3):228–234.

Parry-Fielder B, Nolan TM, Collins KJ, Stojcevski Z. Developmental language disorders and epilepsy. *J. Paediatr. Child Health* 1997; 33(4):277–280.

Patry G, Lyagoubi S, Tassinari A. Subclinical "electrical status epilepticus" induced by sleep in children. *Arch. Neurol.* 1971; 24:242–252.

Paulesu E, Perani D, Blasi V. et al. A functional anatomical model for lip-reading. *J. Neurophysiol.* 2003; 90(3):2005–2013.

Peigneux P, Smith C. Memory processing in relation to sleep. In: Kryger M. (ed.) *Principles and Practice of Sleep Medicine* (5th edn). Elsevier, Philadelphia, 2010; pp. 335–347.

Pera MC, Brazzo D, Altieri N, Balottin U, Veggiotti P. Long-term evolution of neuropsychological competences in encephalopathy with status epilepticus during sleep: A variable prognosis. *Epilepsia* 2013 Oct; 54(Suppl 7):77–85.

Perniola T, Margari L, Buttiglione M, Andreula C, Simone IL, Santostasi R. A case of Landau-Kleffner syndrome secondary to inflammatory demyelinating disease. *Epilepsia* 1993 May–Jun; 34(3):551–556.

Peretz I, Gosselin N, Nan Y, Caron-Caplette E, Trehub SE, Béland R. A novel tool for evaluating children's musical abilities across age and culture. *Front Syst. Neurosci.* 2013 Jul 10; 7:30.

Perniola T, Margari L, Buttiglione M, Andreula C, Simone IL, Santostasi R. A case of Landau-Kleffner syndrome secondary to inflammatory demyelinating disease. *Epilepsia.* 1993 May-Jun; 34(3):551–556.

Peter C, Assal G. Comportement verbal atypique après 30ans d'évolution d'un syndrome d'aphasie-épilepsie acquise. *Psychiatrie de l'enfant.* 1992; XXXXV54(1):109–125.

Picard A, Cheliout Heraut F, Bouskraoui M, Lacert P. Sleep EEG and developmental dysphasia. *Dev. Med. Child Neurol.* 1998; 40(9):595–599.

Piccirilli M, D'Alessandro P, Tiacci C, Ferroni A. Language lateralization in children with benign partial epilepsy. *Epilepsia* 1988; 29(1):19–25.

Plaza M, Rigoard MT, Chevrie-Muller C, Cohen H, Picard A. Short-term memory impairment and unilateral dichotic listening extinction in a child with Landau-Kleffner syndrome: Auditory or phonological disorder? *Brain Cogn.* 2001 Jun–Jul; 46(1–2):235–240.

Platel H, Price C, Baron JC, et al. The structural components of music perception. A functional anatomical study. *Brain* 1997 Feb; 120 (Pt 2):229–243.

Poeppel D, Emmorey K, Hickok G, Pylkkänen L. Towards a new neurobiology of language. *J Neurosci.* 2012 Oct; 32(41):14125–14131.

Poeppel D, Hickok G. Towards a new functional anatomy of language. *Cognition.* 2004 May-Jun; 92(1–2):1–12.

Poizner H, Klima ES, Bellugi U. *What the Hands Reveal about the Brain.* MIT Press, Cambridge, 1987.

Pötzl O. Uber sensorische aphasie in Kindesalter. *Zschr. Hals. Nas. Ohr. hk.* 1926; 14:191–216.

Praline J, Barthez MA, Castelnau P,et al. A typical language impairment in two siblings: relationship with electrical status epilepticus during slow wave sleep. *J Neurol Sci.* 2006 Nov; 249(2):166–171.

Praline J, Hommet C, Barthez MA, et al. Outcome at adulthood of the continuous spike-waves during sleep and Landau-Kleffner syndromes. *Epilepsia* 2003 Nov; 44(11):1434–1440.

Prats JM, Garaizar C, Garcia-Nieto ML, Madoz P. Antiepileptic drugs and atypical evolution of idiopathic partial epilepsy. *Pediatr. Neurol.* 1998; 18(5):402–406.

Prats JM, Garaizar C, Garcia-Nieto ML, Madoz P. Opercular epileptic syndrome: An unusual form of benign partial epilepsy in childhood. *Rev. Neurol.* 1999; 29(4):375–380.

Pressler RM, Binnie CD, Coleshill SG, Chorley GA, Robinson RO. Effect of lamotrigine on cognition in children with epilepsy. *Neurology* 23 May 2006; 66(10):1495–1499.

Pressler RM, Brandl U. Transitory cognitive impairment during very brief subclinical EEG discharges in children. *Epilepsia* 1995; 36(Suppl 3):A93.

Pressler RM, Robinson RO, Wilson GA, Binnie CD. Treatment of interictal epileptiform discharges can improve behavior in children with behavioral problems and epilepsy. *J. Pediatr.* 2005 Jan; 146(1):112–117.

Pullens P, Pullens W, Blau V, Sorger B, Jansma BM, Goebel R. Evidence for normal letter-sound integration, but altered language pathways in a case of recovered Landau-Kleffner Syndrome. *Brain Cogn.* 2015 Oct; 99:32–45.

Raichle ME. The brain's default mode network. *Annu. Rev. Neurosci.* 2015; 38:433–447.

Rapin I. Dementia Infantilis (Heller's dementia). In Carter CH. (ed.) *Medical Aspects of Mental Retardation.* CC Thomas, Springfield, IL, 1965.

Rapin I. Verbal auditory agnosia, Letter to The Editor, *Dev. Med. Child Neurol.* 1988; 3.

Rapin I. Autistic children: Diagnosis and clinical features. *Pediatrics* 1991; 87:751–760.

Rapin I. Autistic regression and disintegrative disorder: how important the role of epilepsy? *Semin Pediatr Neurol.* 1995 Dec; 2(4):278–285.

Rapin I. Reply to Woll and Sieratzki. *J. Child Neurol.* 1996; 11:848–849.

Rapin I, Allen DA. Syndromes in developmental and adult aphasia. *Res. Publ. Assoc. Res. Nerv. Ment. Dis.* 1988; 66:57–75.

Rapin I, Mattis S, Rowan AJ, Golden GG. Verbal auditory agnosia in children. *Dev. Med. Child Neurol.* 1977; 19:192–207.

Rating D, Wolf C, Bast T. Sulthiame as monotherapy in children with benign childhood epilepsy with centrotemporal spikes: A 6-month randomized, double-blind, placebo- controlled study. Sulthiame study group. *Epilepsia* 2000; 41(10):1284–1288.

Rejnö-Habte Selassie G, Hedström A, Viggedal G, Jennische M, Kyllerman M. Speech, language, and cognitive dysfunction in children with focal epileptiform activity: A follow-up study. *Epilepsy Behav.* 2010; 18(3):267–275.

Reutlinger C, Helbig I, Gawelczyk B, et al. Deletions in 16p13 including GRIN2A in patients with intellectual disability, various dysmorphic features, and seizure disorders of the rolandic region. *Epilepsia* 2010 Sep; 51(9):1870–1873.

Riedner BA, Vyazovskiy VV, Huber R, et al. Sleep homeostasis and cortical synchronization: III. A high-density EEG study of sleep slow waves in humans. *Sleep* 2007 Dec; 30(12):1643–1657.

Ripley K, Lea J. *A Follow-Up Study of Receptive Aphasic Ex-Pupils.* Printed by Promotion House Limited, Edenbridge, Kent, UK, 1984.

Robinson RO, Baird G, Robinson G, Simonoff E. Landau-Kleffner syndrome: Course and correlates with outcome. *Dev. Med. Child. Neurol.* 2001; 43:243–247.

Roll P, Rudolf G, Pereira S, et al. SRPX2 mutations in disorders of language cortex and cognition. *Hum. Mol. Genet.* 1 Apr 2006; 15(7):1195–1207.

Rossi PG, Parmeggiani A, Posar A, Scaduto MC, Chiodo S, Vatti G. Landau-Kleffner syndrome (LKS): Long-term follow-up and links with electrical status epilepticus during sleep (ESES). *Brain Dev.* 1999; 21:90–98.

Roubertie A, Humbertclaude V, Rivier F, Cheminal R, Echenne B. Interictal paroxysmal epileptic discharges during sleep in childhood: Phenotypic variability in a family. *Epilepsia* 2003; 44(6):864–869.

Roulet-Perez E, Deonna T. Autism, epilepsy and EEG epileptiform activity In. Autism: A neurological disorder of early brain development. International Child Neurology Association MacKeith Press, 2006; 174–188.

Roulet-Perez E, Deonna T, Despland PA. Prolonged intermittent drooling and oromotor dyspraxia in benign childhood epilepsy with centrotemporal spikes. *Epilepsia* 1989; 30(5):564–568.

Roulet-Perez E, Deonna T, Gaillard F, Peter-Favre C, Despland PA. Acquired aphasia, dementia and behavior disorder with epilepsy and continuous spike and waves during sleep in a child. *Epilepsia* 1991; 32(4):495–503.

Roulet-Perez E. Syndromes of acquired apileptic aphasia and epilepsy with continuous spike-wave discharges during sleep model of prolonged cognitive impairment of epileptic origin. *Sem. Pediatr. Neurol.* 1995; 2:269–277.

Roulet-Perez E, Davidoff V, Despland PA, Deonna T. Mental and behavioural deterioration of children with epilepsy and CSWS: Acquired epileptic frontal syndrome. *Dev. Med. Child Neurol.* 1993; 35:661–674.

Roulet-Perez E, Davidoff V, Prélaz AC, et al. Sign language in childhood epileptic aphasia (Landau-Kleffner syndrome). *Dev. Med. Child Neurol.* 2001; 43(11):739–744.

Roulet-Perez E, Maeder P, Villemure KM, Chaves Vischer V, Villemure JG. Acquired hippocampal damage after temporal lobe seizures in 2 infants. *Ann. Neurol.* 2000; 48:384–387.

Roulet-Perez E, Mayor C, Davidoff V, et al. Dymanics of development before and after early epilepsy surgery: Sorting out the direct effects of epilepsy. Abstract. *Eur. J. Paediatr. Neurol.* 2003; 7(5):345–346.

Roulet Perez E, Mayor C, Davidoff V, et al. Dynamics of develoment before and after early epilepsy surgery: sorting out the direct effects of epilepsy. *Epilepsia* 2010; 51(7):1266–1276.

References

Roulet-Perez E, Seek M, Mayer E, Despland PA, De Tribolet N, Deonna T. Childhood epilepsy with neuropschychological regression and continuous spike waves during sleep: Epilepsy surgery in a young adult. *Eur. J. Paediatr. Neurol.* 1998; 2:303–311.

Roulet-Perez E. Langue des signes et langue parlée: Compétition ou synergie? *Paediatrica* 2001; 37–40.

Rubboli G, Tassinari CA. Negative myoclonus. An overview of its clinical features, pathophysiological mechanisms, and management. *Neurophysiol. Clin.* 2006 Sep–Dec; 36(5–6):337–343.

Sacks O. *Seeing Voices*. Picador, London, 1991.

Sacks O. *Musicophilia: Tales of music and the brain,* New York: Alfred A. Knopf, 2007.

Saito K, Otsuki M, Ueno S. Sign language aphasia due to a left occipital lesion in a deaf signer. *Neurology.* 2007 Oct; 69(14):1466–1468.

Saltik S, Uluduz D, Cokar O, Demirbilek V, Dervent A. A clinical and EEG study on idiopathic partial epilepsies with evolution into ESES spectrum disorders. *Epilepsia* 2005 Apr; 46(4):524–533.

Sánchez Fernández I, Loddenkemper T. Pediatric focal epilepsy syndromes. *J. Clin. Neurophysiol.* 2012 Oct; 29(5):425–440.

Sánchez Fernández I, Loddenkemper T, Galanopoulou AS, Moshé SL. Should epileptiform discharges be treated? *Epilepsia* 2015 Oct; 56(10):1492–1504.

Sanchez Fernández IS, Peters JM, Hadjiloizou S, et al. Clinical staging and electroencephalographic evolution of continuous spikes and waves during sleep. *Epilepsia* 2012a Jul; 53(7):1185–1195.

Sánchez Fernández I, Takeoka M, Tas E, et al. Early thalamic lesions in patients with sleep-potentiated epileptiform activity. *Neurology* 29 May 2012b; 78(22):1721–1727.

Sakai KL, Tatsuno Y, Suzuki K, Kimura H, Ichida Y. Sign and speech: Amodal commonality in left hemisphere dominance for comprehension of sentences. *Brain* 2005 Jun; 128(Pt 6):1407–1417.

Sarco DP, Boyer K, Lundy-Krigbaum SM, et al. Benign rolandic epileptiform discharges are associated with mood and behavior problems. *Epilepsy Behav.* 2011 Oct; 22(2):298–303.

Scheltens-de Boer M. Guidelines for EEG in encephalopathy related to ESES/CSWS in children. *Epilepsia* 2009 Aug; 50(Suppl 7):13–17.

Scheffer IE, Heron SE, Regan BM, et al. Mutations in mammalian target of rapamycin regulator DEPDC5 cause focal epilepsy with brain malformations. *Ann. Neurol.* 2014 May; 75(5):782–787.

Scheffer IE, Jones L, Pozzebon M, Howel A, Saling M, Berkovic SF. Autosomal dominant rolandic epilepsy and speech dyspraxia: A new syndrome with anticipation *Ann. Neurol.* 1995; 38:633–664.

Scholtes FB, Hendriks MP, Renier WO. Cognitive deterioration and electrical status epilepticus during slow sleep. *Epilepsy Behav.* 2005 Mar; 6(2):167–173.

Schneebaum-Sender N, Goldberg-Stern H, Fattal-Valevski A, Kramer U. Does a normalizing electroencephalogram in benign childhood epilepsy with centrotemporal spikes abort attention deficit hyperactivity disorder? *Pediatr. Neurol.* 2012 Oct; 47(4):279–283.

Schwartz TH, Bonhoeffer T. In vivo optical mapping of epileptic foci and surround inhibition in ferret cerebral cortex. *Nat. Med.* 2001 Sep; 7(9):1063–1067.

Scott SK, McGettigan C, Eisner F. A little more conversation, a little less action – Candidate roles for the motor cortex in speech perception. *Nat. Rev. Neurosci.* 2009 Apr; 10(4):295–302.

Seegmüller C, Deonna T, Dubois CM, et al. Long-term outcome after cognitive and behavioral regression in nonlesional epilepsy with continuous spike-waves during slow-wave sleep. *Epilepsia* 2012 Jun; 53(6):1067–1076.

Seibert JM, Hogan AE, Mundy PC. Assessing interactional competencies: The early social-communication scale. *Infant Ment. Health J.* 1982; 3:244–258.

Seri S, Cerquiglini A, Pisani F. Spike-induced interference in auditory sensory processing in Landau-Kleffner syndrome. *Electroencephalogr. Clin. Neurophysiol.* 1998; 108(5):506–510.

Shafrir Y, Prensky AL. Acquired epileptiform opercular syndrrome: A second case report, review of the literature, and comparison to the Landau-Kleffner syndrome. *Epilepsia* 1995; 36(10):1050–1057.

Shamdeen MG, Jost W, Frohnhöfer M, Gortner L, Meyer S. Effect of sulthiame on EEG pathology, behavior and school performance in children with rolandic epileptiform discharges. *Pediatr. Int.* 2012 Dec; 54(6):798–800.

Shewmon DA, Erwin RJ. Focal spike-induced cerebral dysfunction is related to the after-coming slow wave. *Ann. Neurol.* 1988; 23:131–137.

Shewmon DA, Erwin RJ. Transient visual impairment of visual perception induced by simple interictal occipital spikes. *J. Clin. Exp. Neuropsychol.* 1989; 4(5):675–691.

Shinnar S, Rapin I, Tuchman RF, et al. Language regression in childhood. *Pediatr. Neurol.* 2001; 24(3):183–189.

Shuper A, Stahl B, Mimouni M. Transient opercular syndrome: a manifestation of uncontrolled epileptic activity. *Acta Neurol Scand.* 2000 May; 101(5):335–338.

Sieratzki JS, Calvert GA, Brammer M, David A, Woll B. Accessibility of spoken, written, and sign language in Landau-Kleffner syndrome: A linguistic and functional MRI study. *Epileptic Disord.* 2001 Jun; 3(2):79–89.

Sinclair DB, Snyder TJ. Corticosteroids for the treatment of Landau-Kleffner syndrome and continuous spike-wave discharge during sleep. *Pediatr. Neurol.* 2005 May; 32(5):300–306.

Siniatchkin M, Groening K, Moehring J, et al. Neuronal networks in children with continuous spikes and waves during slow sleep. *Brain* 2010; 133:2798–2813.

Smith AB, Kavros PM, Clarke T, Dorta NJ, Tremont G, Pal DK. A neurocognitive endophenotype associated with rolandic epilepsy. *Epilepsia* 2012 Apr; 53(4):705–711.

Smith MC, Pierre-Louis SJ, Kanner A, et al. Pathological spectrum of acquired epileptic aphasia of childhood. Abstract *Epilepsia* 1992; 33(Suppl 3):p.115.

Solomon G, Carson D, Pavlakis S, Fraser R, Labar D. Intracranial Monitoring in Landau-Kleffner syndrome Associated with Left Temporal Lobe Astrocytoma. *Epilepsia* 1993; 34(3):557–560.

Spanaki MV, Kopylev L, DeCarli C, et al. Postoperative changes in cerebral metabolism in temporal lobe epilepsy. *Arch. Neurol.* 2000; 57:1447–1452.

Spilrein S. Quelques analogies entre la pensée de l'enfant, celle de la pensée et l'aphasique Subconscient. *Arch. Psychol.* 1923; 18:306–322.

Staden UE, Isaacs E, Boyd SG, Brandl U, Neville BGR. Language dysfunction in children with rolandic epilepsy. *Neuropediatrics* 1998; 29:242–248.

Stefanatos G. Changing perspectives on Landau-Kleffner syndrome. *Clin. Neuropsychol.* 2011 Aug; 25(6):963–988.

Stefanatos GA, Grover W, Geller E. Case study: Corticosteroid treatment of language regression in pervasive developmental disorder. *J. Am. Acad. Child Adolesc. Psychiatry* 1995; 34:1107–1111.

Stefanatos GA, Kinsbourne M, Wasserstein J. Acquired epileptiform aphasia: A dimensional view of Landau-Kleffner syndrome and the relation to regressive autistic spectrum disorders. *Child Neuropsychol.* 2002; 8(3):195–228.

Stein LK Curry FKW. Childhood auditory agnosia. *J. Speech Hear. Disord.* 33(4).

Steriade M, Contreras D. Spike-wave complexes and fast component of cortically generated seizures. I Role of neocortex and thalamus. *J Neurophysiol.* 1998; 80:1439–1455.

Suleiman J, Dale RC. The recognition and treatment of autoimmune epilepsy in children. *Dev Med Child Neurol.* 2015 May; 57(5):431–440.

Suleiman J, Wright S, Gill D, et al. Autoantibodies to neuronal antigens in children with new-onset seizures classified according to the revised ILAE organization of seizures and epilepsies. *Epilepsia* 2013 Dec; 54(12):2091–2100.

Szabó L, Nagy J, Kálmánchey R. Adrenocorticotropic hormone therapy in acquired childhood epileptic aphasia. *Ideggyogy Sz.* 30 Nov 2008; 61(11–12):409–416.

Tachikawa E, Oguni H, Shirakawa S, Funatsuka M, Hayashi K, Osawa M. Acquired epileptiform opercular syndrome: A case report and results of single photon emission computed tomography and computer-assisted electroencephalographic analysis. *Brain Dev.* 2001 Jul; 23(4):246–250.

Takeoka M, Riviello JJ Jr, Duffy FH, et al. Bilateral volume reduction of the superior temporal areas in Landau-Kleffner syndrome. *Neurology* 12 Oct 2004; 63(7):1289–1292.

Tankus A, Fried I, Shoham S. Structured neuronal encoding and decoding of human speech features. *Nat. Comm.* 2012; 3:1–3.

Tassinari CA, Cantalupo G, Rios-Pohl L, Giustina ED, Rubboli G. Encephalopathy with status epilepticus during slow sleep: "The Penelope syndrome". *Epilepsia* 2009 Aug; 50(Suppl 7):4–8.

Tassinari CA, Rubboli G, Volpi L, Billard C, Bureau M. In *Les Syndromes Epileptiques de l'enfant et de l'adolescent* (eds J. Roger, et al.). John Libbey Eurotext, 2002; pp. 265–283.

Tassinari CA, Rubboli G, Volpi L, et al. Encephalopathy with electrical status epilepticus during slow sleep or ESES syndrome including the acquired aphasia. *Clin. Neurophysiol.* 2000 Sep; 111(Suppl 2):S94–S102.

Television Suisse Romande (TSR). La langue des signes au service des autres. Television Series: "Signes" (program for the deaf community in sign language), 2005.

Tepmongkol S, Srikijvilaikul T, Vasavid P. Factors affecting bilateral temporal lobe hypometabolism on 18F-FDG PET brain scan in unilateral medial temporal lobe epilepsy. *Epilepsy Behav.* 2013; 29:386–389.

Tesfaye N, Seaquist ER, Oz G. Noninvasive measurement of brain glycogen by nuclear magnetic resonance spectroscopy and its application to the study of brain metabolism. *J. Neurosci. Res.* 2011; 89:1905–1912.

Tohyama J, Akasaka N, Ohashi T, Kobayashi Y. Acquired opercular epilepsy with oromotor dysfunction: Magnetoencephalographic analysis and efficacy of corticosteroid therapy. *J. Child Neurol.* 2011 Jul; 26(7):885–890.

References

Tononi G, Cirelli C. Sleep and synaptic homeostasis: A hypothesis. *Brain Res. Bull.* 2003 Dec 15; 62(2):143–150.

Tononi G, Cirelli C. Sleep and the price of plasticity: From synaptic and cellular homeostasis to memory consolidation and integration. *Neuron* 2014 Jan 8; 81(1):12–34.

Tovia E, Goldberg-Stern H, Ben Zeev B, et al. The prevalence of atypical presentations and comorbidities of benign childhood epilepsy with centrotemporal spikes. *Epilepsia* 2011 Aug; 52(8):1483–1488.

Tsai MH, Vears DF, Turner SJ, et al. Clinical genetic study of the epilepsy-aphasia spectrum. *Epilepsia* 2013 Feb; 54(2):280–287.

Tsuru T, Mori M, Mizuguchi M, Momoi MY. Effects of high-dose intravenous corticosteroid therapy in Landau-Kleffner syndrome. *Pediatr. Neurol.* 2000 Feb; 22(2):145–147.

Tuchman R. Treatment of seizure disorders and EEG abnormalities in children with autism spectrum disorders. *J. Autism Dev. Disord.* 2000; 30(5):485–489.

Tuchman RF. Regression in pervasive developmental disorders: Is there a relationship with Laudau-Kleffner syndrome? *Ann. Neurol.* 1995; 38:526.

Tuchman R, Rapin I. Regression in pervasive developmental disorders: Seizures and epileptiform electroencephalographic correlates. *Pediatrics.* 1997; 99:560–566.

Tuchman R, Rapin I. Epilepsy in autism. *Lancet Neurol.* 2002; 1(6):352–358.

Tuchman RF, Rapin I, Shinnar S. Autistic and dysphasic children. I: Clinical characteristics. *Pediatrics.* 1991 Dec; 88(6):1211–1218.

Tuchman RF, Rapin I, Shinnar S. Autistic and dysphasic children. II: Epilepsy. *Pediatrics.* 1991; 88:1219–1225.

Turner SJ, Mayes AK, Verhoeven A, Mandelstam SA, Morgan AT, Scheffer IE. GRIN2A: An aptly named gene for speech dysfunction. *Neurology* 10 Feb 2015a; 84(6):586–593.

Turner SJ, Morgan AT, Perez ER, Scheffer IE. New genes for focal epilepsies with speech and language disorders. *Curr. Neurol. Neurosci. Rep.* 2015b Jun; 15(6):35. doi:10.1007/s11910-015-0554-0. Erratum in: *Curr. Neurol. Neurosci. Rep.* 2015 Aug; 15(8):55.

Uldall P, Sahlholdt L, Alving J. Landau-Kleffner syndrome with onset at 18 months and an initial diagnosis of pervasive developmental disorder. *Eur. J. Paediatr. Neurol.* 2000; 4:81–86.

Uliel-Sibony S, Kramer U. Benign childhood epilepsy with centro-temporal spikes (BCECTSs), electrical status epilepticus in sleep (ESES), and academic decline – How aggressive should we be? *Epilepsy Behav.* 2015 Mar; 44:117–120.

Urbain C, Di Vincenzo T, Peigneux P, Van Bogaert P. Is sleep-related consolidation impaired in focal idiopathic epilepsies of childhood? A pilot study. *Epilepsy Behav.* 2011 Oct; 22(2):380–384.

Vadlamudi L, Harvey AS, Connellan MM, et al. Is benign rolandic epilepsy genetically determined? *Ann. Neurol.* 2004 Jul; 56(1):129–132.

Vadlamudi L, Kjeldsen MJ, Corey LA, et al. Analyzing the aetiology of benign rolandic epilepsy: A multicenter twin collaboration. *Epilepsia* 2006 Mar; 47(3):550–555.

Van Bogaert P. Epileptic encephalopathy with continuous spike-waves during slow-wave sleep including Landau-Kleffner syndrome. *Handb. Clin. Neurol.* 2013; 111:635–640.

Van Bogaert P, King MD, Paquier P, et al. Acquired auditory agnosia in childhood and normal sleep electroencephalography subsequently diagnosed as Landau-Kleffner syndrome: A report of three cases. *Dev. Med. Child Neurol.* 2013 Jun; 55(6):575–579.

Van Bogaert P, Wikler D, Damhaut P, Szliwowski HB, Goldman S. Regional changes in glucose metabolism during brain development from the age of 6 years. *Neuroimage* 1998a; 8:62–68.

Van Bogaert P, Wikler D, Damhaut P, Szliwowski HB, Goldman S. Cerebral glucose metabolism and centrotemporal spikes. *Epilepsy Res.* 1998b; 29:123–127.

Van Bogaert P, Massager N, Tugendhaft P, et al. Statistical parametric mapping of regional glucose metabolism in mesial temporal lobe epilepsy. *Neuroimage* 2000; 12:129–138.

Van Bogaert P, Aeby A, De Borchgrave V, et al. The epileptic syndromes with continuous spikes and waves during slow sleep: Definition and management guidelines. *Acta Neurol. Belg.* 2006; 106:52–60.

Van Bogaert P, Urbain C, Galer S, Ligot N, Peigneux P, De Tiège X. Impact of focal interictal epileptiform discharges on behaviour and cognition in children. *Neurophysiol. Clin.* 2012; 42:53–58.

Van den Munckhof B, van Dee V, Sagi L, et al. Treatment of electrical status epilepticus in sleep: A pooled analysis of 575 cases. *Epilepsia* 2015 Nov; 56(11):1738–1746.

Van Landingham KE, Lothman EW. Self-sustaining limbic status epilepticus. I. Acute and chronic cerebral metabolic studies: Limbic hypermetabolism and neocortical hypometabolism. *Neurology* 1991; 41:1942–1949.

Van Paesschen W, Dupont P, Van Driel G, Van Billoen H, Maes A. SPECT perfusion changes during complex partial seizures in patients with hippocampal sclerosis. *Brain* 2003; 126:1103–1111.

Van Paesschen W, Porke K, Fannes K, et al. Cognitive deficits during status epilepticus and time course of recovery: A case report. *Epilepsia* 2007; 48:1979–1983.

Vance M. Educational and therapeutic approaches used with a child presenting with acquired aphasia with convulsive disorder (Landau-Kleffner syndrome). *Child Lang. Teach. Ther.* 1991; 7:41–60.

Vance M. Christopher Lumpship: Developing phonological representations in a child with auditory processing deficit. In: Chiat S, Law J, Marshall J. (eds.) *Language Disorders in Children and Adults: Psycholinguistic Approaches to Therapy.* Whurr Publishers, London, 2001; pp. 17–41.

Vanderlinden L, Ceulemans B, Boel M, Van Coster R, Lagae L. Thalamic lesions and epilepsy with continuous spike-waves during slow sleep: A recognizable syndrome. *Eur. J. Paediatr. Neurol.* 2003; 7(5):328.

Vannest J, Tenney JR, Gelineau-Morel R, Maloney T, Glauser TA. Cognitive and behavioral outcomes in benign childhood epilepsy with centrotemporal spikes. *Epilepsy Behav.* 2015 Apr; 45:85–91.

Vears DF, Tsai MH, Sadleir LG, et al. Clinical genetic studies in benign childhood epilepsy with centrotemporal spikes. *Epilepsia* 2012 Feb; 53(2):319–324.

Veggiotti P, Beccaria F, Guerrini R, Capovilla G, Lanzi, G. Continuous spike- and-wave activity during slow-wave sleep: Syndrome or EEG pattern? *Epilepsia* 1999; 40(11):1593–1601.

Veggiotti P, Beccaria F, Papalia G, Termine C, Piazza F, Lanzi G. Continuous spikes and waves during sleep in children with shunted hydrocephalus. *Child's Nerv. Syst.* 1998, 14:188–194.

Veggiotti P, Bova S, Granocchio E, Papalia G, Termine C, Lanzi G. Acquired epileptic frontal syndrome as long-term outcome in two children with CSWS. *Neurophysiol. Clin.* 2001; 31(6):387–397.

Veggiotti P, Pera MC, Teutonico F, Brazzo D, Balottin U, Tassinari CA. Therapy of encephalopathy with status epilepticus during sleep (ESES/CSWS syndrome): An update. *Epileptic Disord.* 2012 Mar; 14(1):1–11.

Verrotti A, Filippini M, Matricardi S, Agostinelli MF, Gobbi G. Memory impairment and Benign Epilepsy with centrotemporal spike(BECTS): A growing suspicion. *Brain Cogn.* 2014 Feb; 84(1):123–131.

Verrotti A, Matricardi S, Di Giacomo DL, Rapino D, Chiarelli F, Coppola G. Neuropsychological impairment in children with Rolandic epilepsy and in their siblings. *Epilepsy Behav.* 2013 Jul; 28(1):108–112.

Vezzani A, French J, Bartfai T, Baram TZ. The role of inflammation in epilepsy. *Nat Rev Neurol.* 2011 Jan;7(1):31–40

Vigevano F, Specchio N, Fejerman N. Idiopathic focal epilepsies. *Handb. Clin. Neurol.* 2013; 111:591–604.

Westphal A, Schelinski S, Volkmar F, Pelphrey K. Revisiting regression in autism: Heller's dementia infantilis. Includes a translation of Über Dementia Infantilis. *J Autism Dev Disord.* 2013 Feb; 43(2):265–271.

Winawer MR, Ottman R, Hauser WA, Pedley TA. Autosomal dominant partial epilepsy with auditory features: Defining the phenotype. *Neurology* 13 Jun 2000; 54(11):2173–2176.

Wioland N, Rudolf G, Metz-Lutz MN. Electrophysiological evidence of persisting unilateral auditory cortex dysfunction in the late outcome of Landau and Kleffner syndrome. *Clin. Neurophysiol.* 2001; 112:319–323.

Wirrell E, Sherman EM, Vanmastrigt R, Hamiwka L. Deterioration in cognitive function in children with benign epilepsy of childhood with central temporal spikes treated with sulthiame. *J. Child Neurol.* 2008 Jan; 23(1):14–21.

Witte OW, Bruehl C. Distant functional and metabolic disturbances in focal epilepsy. *Adv. Neurol.* 1999; 81:383–388.

Wolff M, Weiskopf N, Serra E, Preissl H, Birbaumer N, Kraegeloh-Mann I. Benign partial epilepsy in childhood: Selective cognitive deficits are related to the location of focal spikes determined by combined EEG/MEG. *Epilepsia* 2005 Oct; 46(10):1661–1667.

Worster-Drought C. An unusual form of acquired aphasia in children. *Dev. Med. Child Neurol.* 1971 Oct; 13(5):563–571.

Wuerfel E, Bien CG, Vincent A, Woodhall M, Brockmann K. Glycine receptor antibodies in a boy with focal epilepsy and episodic behavioral disorder. *J. Neurol. Sci.* 2014 Aug 15; 343(1–2):180–182.

Yung AWY, Park YD, Cohen MJ, Garrison TN. Cognitive and behavioral problems in children with centrotemporal spikes. *Pediatr. Neurol.* 2000; 23(5):391–395.

Zaiwalla Z, Stores G. Case reports. In: Beaumanoir A, Bureau A, Deonna T, Mira C, Tassinari CA. (eds) *Continuous Spike and Waves During Slow Sleep, Electrical Status Epilepticus during Slow Sleep. Mariani Foundation Neurology Series: 3.* John Libbey, London, pp. 196–199.

Zappella M. Autistic regression with and without EEG abnormalities followed by favourable outcome. *Brain Dev.* 2010 Oct; 32(9):739–745.

Zardini G, Molteni B, Nardocci N. Linguistic development in a patient with Landau-Kleffner syndrome: A nine year follow up. *Neuropediatrics* 1995; 26:19–25.

INDEX

Recent titles from Mac Keith Press www.mackeith.co.uk

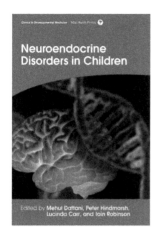

Neuroendocrine Disorders in Children
Mehul Dattani, Peter Hindmarsh, Lucinda Carr and Iain Robinson (Editors)

Clinics in Developmental Medicine
November 2016 ▪ 422pp ▪ hardback ▪ 978-1-909962-50-7
£74.95/ €93.70/ $120.00

Impairments in the interaction between the central nervous system and the endocrine system can lead to a number of disorders in children. These include type 1 diabetes, growth disorders, adrenal thyroid and pituitary problems, Addison's disease and Cushing syndrome, among others. *Neuroendocrine Disorders in Children* provides a comprehensive examination of paediatric and adolescent disorders focusing on the basic science and its clinical relevance.

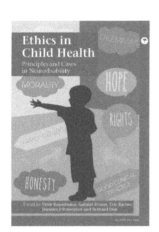

Ethics in Child Health: Principles and Cases in Neurodisability
Peter L. Rosenbaum, Gabriel M. Ronen, Eric Racine, Jennifer Johannesen and Bernard Dan (Editors)

2016 ▪ 396pp ▪ softback ▪ 978-1-909962-63-7
£39.95 / €50.00 / $60.00

This book explores the ethical dimensions of issues that have either been ignored or not recognised. Each chapter is built around an illustrative scenario and discusses how ethical principles can be utilised to inform decision-making. 'Themes for Discussion' at the end of each chapter will help professionals and policy makers put practical ethical thinking at the heart of care.

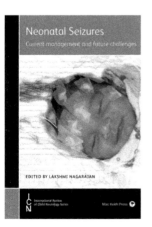

Neonatal Seizures: Current Management and Future Challenges
Lakshmi Nagarajan (Editor)

International Review of Child Neurology Series
2016 ▪ 214pp ▪ hardback ▪ 978-1-909962-67-5
£44.99 / €58.40 / $65.00

This book distils what is known about the many advances in the management of neonatal seizures into one scholarly yet practical text. Chapters cover the neonatal neuron, the use of video EEG in diagnosis, advances in neurophysiology, genetics and neuroprotective strategies, as well as outcomes. This volume will be of use to neonatologists, paediatricians, neurologists and all health professionals involved in the care of neonates experiencing seizures.

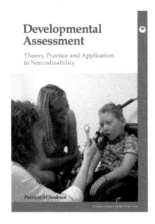

Developmental Assessment: Theory, Practice and Application to Neurodisability
Patricia M. Sonksen

A practical guide from Mac Keith Press
2016 ▪ 384pp ▪ softback ▪ 978-1-909962-56-9
£39.95 / €56.50 / $65.00

This handbook presents a new approach to assessing development in preschool children that can be applied across the developmental spectrum. The reader is taught how to confirm whether development is typical, and if it is not, is signposted to the likely nature and severity of the impairments with a plan of action. The author uses numerous case vignettes from her 40 years' experience to bring to life her approach with clear summary key points and helpful illustrations.

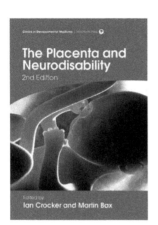

The Placenta and Neurodisability, 2nd Edition
Ian Crocker and Martin Bax (Editors)

Clinics in Developmental Medicine
2015 ▪ 176pp ▪ hardback ▪ 978-1-909962-53-8
£50.00 / €67.50 / $80.00

This comprehensive and authoritative book discusses the critical role of the utero-placenta in neurodisability, both at term and preterm. It examines aspects of fetal compromise and possible cerebro-protective interventions, recent evidence on fetal growth and mental illness, as well as cerebro-therapeutics. Throughout the book, information from the basic sciences is placed within the clinical context.

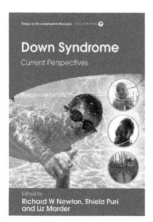

Down Syndrome: Current Perspectives
Richard W. Newton, Shiela Puri and Liz Marder (Editors)

Clinics in Developmental Medicine
2015 ▪ 320pp ▪ hardback ▪ 978-1-909962-47-7
£95.00 / €128.30 / $150.00

Down syndrome remains the most common recognisable form of intellectual disability. The challenge for doctors today is how to capture the rapidly expanding body of scientific knowledge and devise models of care to meet the needs of individuals and their families. *Down Syndrome: Current Perspectives* provides doctors and other health professionals with the information they need to address the challenges that can present in the management of this syndrome.